Register Now for Online Access to Your Book!

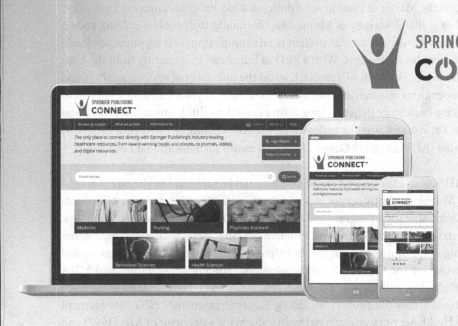

SPRINGER PUBLISHING CONNECT™

Your print purchase of *Applied Problem-Solving in Healthcare Management*, **includes online access to the contents of your book**—increasing accessibility, portability, and searchability!

Access today at:
http://connect.springerpub.com/content/book/978-0-8261-6565-7
or scan the QR code at the right with your smartphone
and enter the access code below.

8BYE3E6L

Scan here for quick access.

SPRINGER PUBLISHING
View all our products at springerpub.com

Sandra J. Potthoff, PhD, is a retired professor from the University of South Florida, Tampa, where she served as the Chair of the Department of Health Policy and Management. She was previously associate professor and is now emeritus associate professor at the University of Minnesota, where she served as the Master of Healthcare Administration Program Director for 8 years. While a faculty member at the University of Minnesota, she taught the problem-solving course for 15 years, and served as a faculty advisor for student teams completing their capstone advanced problem-solving course for almost 25 years. With a PhD in Industrial Engineering from the University of Wisconsin-Madison, Dr. Potthoff's research spans the interfaces of systems analysis and quality management, operations research and management science, and data analytics, applied to evaluating and improving healthcare delivery, long-term care, telehealth homecare services, and community programs. Dr. Potthoff was the recipient of the Association of University Programs in Health Administration (AUPHA) 2019 Gary L. Filerman award for Educational Leadership.

Justine H. Mishek, MHA, is an experienced graduate education lecturer and healthcare management consultant. Ms. Mishek currently serves as senior lecturer for the University of Minnesota Master of Healthcare Administration Program and is a part of the Program Leadership Team. Ms. Mishek is the lead instructor for the Minnesota Problem-Solving Method curriculum, teaches Strategy and Marketing curriculum for both the full-time and executive MHA programs, and assists as a faculty advisor for the CLARION interprofessional student organization and MHA student case competitions. Ms. Mishek has extensive healthcare management experience from prior leadership positions across the country including Kaiser Permanente, ECG Management Consultants, Fairview Health Services, and athenaHealth. She holds a Bachelor of Arts (1997) and a Master of Healthcare Administration (2002) degree from the University of Minnesota. In 2019, Ms. Mishek received the University of Minnesota School of Public Health's Charles N. Hewitt Creative Teaching Award.

Gregory W. Hart, MHA, is a principal with CliftonLarsenAllen (CLA), where he serves in the healthcare consulting practice, and an alumnus of the University of Minnesota MHA Program. Mr. Hart has more than 40 years of experience in healthcare leadership and management. Before joining CLA in 1995 he served as CEO for the University of Minnesota Health System, an academic medical center. He focuses his professional activities in the areas of strategy, mergers, acquisitions, and affiliations. Mr. Hart is a Senior Fellow at the University of Minnesota School of Public Health. He is an active practitioner instructor in the University of Minnesota's MHA program, and has taught and mentored MHA students in the problem-solving course for over 40 years. In 2018, the Greg Hart Distinguished Service Award was created by the MHA Program and its Alumni Association/Foundation to recognize extraordinary alumni for their sustained and exemplary commitment to the MHA Program, its student body, and alumni community. Mr. Hart was honored as its first recipient. He has also twice received the University of Minnesota School of Public Health Community Partner Star Award to recognize his contributions to the education, training, and guidance of the next generation of public health leaders.

APPLIED PROBLEM-SOLVING IN HEALTHCARE MANAGEMENT

Sandra J. Potthoff, PhD

Justine H. Mishek, MHA

Gregory W. Hart, MHA

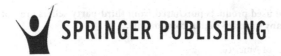 SPRINGER PUBLISHING

Springer Publishing Company, LLC
11 West 42nd Street, New York, NY 10036
www.springerpub.com
connect.springerpub.com/

Acquisitions Editor: David D'Addona
Compositor: Exeter Premedia Services Private Ltd.

Front cover art: Alison P. Sauter, Shelf Studio, Principal and Creative Director, Austin, Texas

ISBN: 978-0-8261-6564-0
e-book ISBN: 978-0-8261-6565-7
DOI: 10.1891/9780826165657

Qualified instructors may request supplements by emailing textbook@springerpub.com
Student resources may be accessed at http://connect.springerpub.com/content/book/978-0-8261-6565-7

Instructor's Manual ISBN: 978-0-8261-6566-4
Sample Syllabus ISBN: 978-0-8261-6567-1
Student Resources ISBN: 978-0-8261-6562-6

20 21 22 23 24 / 5 4 3 2 1

The author and the publisher of this Work have made every effort to use sources believed to be reliable to provide information that is accurate and compatible with the standards generally accepted at the time of publication. The author and publisher shall not be liable for any special, consequential, or exemplary damages resulting, in whole or in part, from the readers' use of, or reliance on, the information contained in this book. The publisher has no responsibility for the persistence or accuracy of URLs for external or third-party Internet websites referred to in this publication and does not guarantee that any content on such websites is, or will remain, accurate or appropriate.

Library of Congress Cataloging-in-Publication Data

Names: Potthoff, Sandra J., author. | Mishek, Justine, author. | Hart,
  Gregory, author.
Title: Applied problem-solving in healthcare management / Sandra J.
  Potthoff, Justine Mishek, Gregory Hart.
Description: First Springer Publishing edition. | New York, NY : Springer
  Publishing Company, LLC, 2021. | Includes bibliographical references and
  index.
Identifiers: LCCN 2020035107 (print) | LCCN 2020035108 (ebook) | ISBN
  9780826165640 (paperback) | ISBN 9780826165657 (ebook)
Subjects: MESH: Health Services Administration | Decision Making,
  Organizational | Organizational Case Studies | Problem Solving
Classification: LCC RA971 (print) | LCC RA971 (ebook) | NLM W 84.1 | DDC
  362.1068--dc23
LC record available at https://lccn.loc.gov/2020035107
LC ebook record available at https://lccn.loc.gov/2020035108

Contact us to receive discount rates on bulk purchases.
We can also customize our books to meet your needs.
For more information please contact: sales@springerpub.com

Sandra Potthoff: https://orcid.org/0000-0001-8602-4625

Publisher's Note: New and used products purchased from third-party sellers are not guaranteed for quality, authenticity, or access to any included digital components.

Printed in the United States of America.

CONTENTS

PART IV: PRACTICE THE ACT PHASE

PART V: PROBLEM-SOLVING CASES

PREFACE

What is the problem?

Who hasn't suffered through yet another unproductive meeting, listening to arguments that seem to be "stuck" when someone at the meeting perceptively asks, "Wait, what's the problem we're trying to solve?"

A problem-solving method taught at the University of Minnesota's Master of Healthcare Administration (MHA) Program since its inception nearly 75 years ago has a way to answer the question, "What is the problem?" and prevent these unproductive meetings from happening. The Problem-Solving Method supports both novices and working professionals in their abilities to discern the complex inter-relationships of problems that face an organization, and in collaboration with the board, the leadership team, and other stakeholders, arrive at a set of action-oriented decisions to move the organization forward. It is comprised of three phases, each of which has several steps: (a) how to DEFINE the problem; (b) how to STUDY the problem; and (c) how to decide upon and implement the best course of ACTION to resolve the problem.

The Problem-Solving Method has been called the "secret sauce" of the Minnesota MHA Program by the students and alumni. It imposes a logical thought process that builds leadership competencies in accurately and effectively defining problems, especially around very complex organizational issues that may involve multiple root causes, and supports arriving at recommendations that get implemented and actually solve the problem at hand. It has withstood the test of time alongside the various trends in quality improvement and consulting tools and methods, such as Lean/Six Sigma, Design Thinking, and Innovation Processes.

As important as the Problem-Solving Method's steps are the "never assume" principles that underlie its use. The Problem-Solving Method requires that you actively listen to and engage with your stakeholders, and that you recognize your own biases and emotions when solving problems. As you practice the Problem-Solving Method, you learn to step outside of yourself, as if you are an external consultant who is unbiased, thoughtful, logical, and empathetic.

This text is a "how-to" guide that describes the Problem-Solving Method in detail. It provides an overview of the method, and step-by-step instructions, tips, tools, activities, and cases to facilitate practicing and learning the Problem-Solving Method. The authors of the text have almost 75 years of experience combined in teaching or advising students in the Problem-Solving Method through case method teaching, problem-solving fieldwork consulting projects, summer residency projects, capstone consulting projects, and case competitions.

The text is especially useful in supporting experiential learning and coaching for students and professionals early in their careers—specifically providing a problem-solving method and tools for students, student teams, and early careerists working with healthcare organizations on consulting projects, or on projects as an administrative intern, resident, or fellow.

For young students and early careerists without much real-world experience, learning the Problem-Solving Method helps them have the confidence to "know how to start a project" in an organization and focus on asking the right questions and developing a scope of work to guide their efforts. The Problem-Solving Method provides a framework to guide them so they can proceed intelligently and independently, without having to rely on the organizational preceptor to provide daily oversight of every project detail. Each major step of the Problem-Solving Method serves as a check-in point for the student and preceptor when discussing the project work underway. The Problem-Solving Method serves as a guide for both parties and builds trust that the project approach will be fruitful and meaningful as well as produce results for the organization.

Experienced healthcare leaders will also find value in this text. The Problem-Solving Method is a disciplined, thorough approach that suppresses making assumptions about the problem and prematurely jumping to solutions. Its steps become an innate cognitive framework that guides evidence-based decision-making, particularly in its approach to defining the problem and engaging stakeholders in the problem-solving process.

The text will assist in facilitating teaching a structured approach to problem-solving and decision-making in undergraduate or graduate level case study, experiential learning, problem-solving and management decision-making courses. Example courses include management courses, internship and residency project courses, capstone project courses, consulting project courses, and case competition courses or preparation. The Problem-Solving Method is applicable whether the situation to which it is being applied is a "real-world" project or a simulated case study in the classroom.

The text will also support teaching leadership and problem-solving skills in early careerist leadership training programs within organizations. In addition, it will be instructive for organizations that wish to enhance the problem-solving and decision making skills of its workforce more broadly.

Within the University of Minnesota MHA Program, teaching the Problem-Solving Method is embedded not only in the case-based problem-solving course, but in the experiential project coursework conducted in healthcare organizations, such as the summer residency and the capstone consulting project course. It is also the methodology used by students as they prepare for case competitions.

We believe healthcare administration programs will find it beneficial to add instruction in teaching the Problem-Solving Method described in this text to their courses that provide credit for case-based and experiential learning efforts. For example, courses that offer credit for summer internships, capstone projects, and case competition participation could adopt the text to teach the Problem-Solving Method as part of the case or project learning. Instructors will find this helpful as not only does it provide a framework that assists students in developing leadership competencies for their success, it also provides a framework and process by which instructors can measure student performance as they look to receive course credit for experiential learning opportunities.

Organizations who adopt the text as part of their administrative fellowship development programs will find benefit in using the Problem-Solving Method as a structured approach to support the success of fellows in developing their ability to excel on their assigned organizational projects. The structure of the method's steps provides natural touchpoints for feedback between the preceptor and the fellow to ensure the fellow is on track. In addition, organizations who adopt the text for leadership workforce development more broadly can use the structure of the cases provided in the text to write organization-specific cases to be used in their training and development activities. This will facilitate active learning by participants in the training that engages them in actually solving the organization's current problems as they apply the Problem-Solving Method in their continuing education.

Sandra J. Potthoff
Justine H. Mishek
Gregory W. Hart

ACKNOWLEDGMENTS

Problem-solving as a leadership and management core competency has been taught in the University of Minnesota Master of Healthcare Administration (MHA) program since its founding in 1946. Alumni of the University of Minnesota's MHA Program have often described the problem-solving course as the "secret sauce" of the program. Many of Minnesota's MHA alumni's most vivid memories of their time in the program revolve around their experiences in the problem-solving course—recommending a novel solution that was implemented by the organization, or experiencing the satisfaction of an effective response to a probing question by a CEO.

The problem-solving course was created and taught by James A. Hamilton, the founder of the Minnesota MHA Program and its director from 1946 until his retirement in 1966. He used a Socratic case method of teaching problem-solving so students could quickly learn how to think and act like healthcare leaders. Hamilton taught the method and placed students in organizations during graduate school in order to ensure Minnesota graduates could accurately diagnose problems and arrive at actionable recommendations that move an organization forward. The students then practiced the method in their year-long internships as they learned how to become administrators under the tutelage of alumni preceptors. The problem-solving process he delineated had fourteen steps:

1. Define the problem by apprehending the real issues of the situation and stating the problem precisely.
2. Budget the time as well as the effort available and necessary to arrive at an acceptable solution.
3. List the areas necessary for consideration to determine the best solution.
4. List the elements to be measured and the best means of measurement.
5. Plan, make contact, collect, and classify data.
6. Make comparisons with others, with existing standards, over past experience.
7. Interpret results of comparisons by seeking the real reasons for variance.
8. Develop temporary conclusions for each element.
9. Consider various solutions; choose the best, not the first acceptable solution.
10. Take a fresh look at the approach to the problem and the selected solution.
11. Develop a plan of accomplishing the solution.

12. Determine recommendations that invite action.

13. Prepare and present a report to those who make the final decision.

14. Implement action to carry out the selected solution.[1(p11)]

The 14 steps of the Problem-Solving Method have evolved over the almost 75 years since the Minnesota MHA Program's inception, although the methodology still relies on these core steps. The evolution has provided more "how-to" detailed steps for novice problem solvers and organized the steps into three phases: define, study, act.

The University of Minnesota MHA's Problem-Solving Method teaches a logical thought process that drives toward identifying all inter-related key issues in a problem, engaging stakeholder input and buy-in, addressing root causes, conducting unbiased research around root causes and alternative solutions, drawing sound conclusions that lead to actionable recommendations, and strategizing on approaches that maximize the probability of acceptance and implementation of the recommendations. Some of our alumni have reported that they have been in national meetings when, as the meeting progressed, they could tell who was a Minnesota alumnus by the way they approached and analyzed the problem at hand.

Hamilton was adamant about creating "boots on the ground" real experiences for his students through internships and residencies—an idea that was not universally endorsed by his peers in education at that time. "My thesis was simple," he said. "You cannot teach a graduate course like hospital administration and have graduates immediately begin to do work of any stature without a practice period."[2(p21)] Hamilton was also a strong believer in having healthcare leaders engaged as preceptors during the students' internship experience. He chose alumni as preceptors who would serve as mentors, teachers, and guides to his students. He called them "hot shots." But even if they were hot shots, Hamilton knew they needed coaching: "You have to be sure you're teaching this…and this…and this!"[2(p21)]

The University of Minnesota MHA program continues Hamilton's methods of case teaching, real-world project experience, and alumni preceptors in teaching problem-solving. For traditional full-time students, the problem-solving course is taught in the second semester of the first year of the curriculum. The method is taught using two written cases and a real-world team project in a healthcare organization under the direction of an alumnus in that organization.

The problem-solving course in the first year of the MHA program prepares students to apply the method in their summer residency to a real-world project agreed upon between the MHA program faculty coordinator and the healthcare organization in which the summer residency occurs. Each student is assigned an alumni summer preceptor outside of the student's host organization to support and reinforce student learning of the method.

In the final semester of their second year, the students apply the method while conducting their capstone course, "Advanced Problem-Solving Projects." Executive students are also taught the University of Minnesota Method of Problem-Solving as they begin the second year of study to apply in their capstone project, other coursework, and their leadership roles in their organizations.

As mentioned, the three authors of this problem-solving field manual collectively have almost 75 years of experience in teaching or advising students in the problem-solving course and the capstone advanced problem-solving course. Prior to us, faculty member Bright Dornblaser and James A. Hamilton's son-in-law, John Sweetland, continued the problem-solving course after Hamilton retired.

The University of Minnesota MHA alumni have collectively dedicated thousands of hours mentoring students in the problem-solving course, the summer residency course, and the capstone course. Students are encouraged to contact alumni across the country as they conduct research for their cases and projects, and the alumni know that they are "required" to return the students' phone calls and emails. Thus, the legacy of never refusing a call from a Minnesota MHA student or alumnus continues. And for that we are forever grateful.

REFERENCES

1. Hamilton JA. *Decision-making in hospital and medical care.* Minneapolis, MN: University of Minnesota Press; 1960.
2. Regents of the University of Minnesota. *Never assume. How an audacious pioneer built the Minnesota MHA Program and why it flourishes today* [Brochure]. Minneapolis, MN: Pine, Carol; 2018. https://indd. adobe.com/view/3234d682-910d-4e22-bab9-a7292b1ed1e0

PROBLEM-SOLVING METHOD TOOLS AND ONLINE STUDENT RESOURCES

The tools and student resources listed below will help you synthesize your work as you use the Problem-Solving Method and move through the textbook. Access the tools and resources online by scanning the QR code or by following this link to Springer Publishing Company Connect™: http://connect.springerpub.com/content/book/978-0-8261-6565-7 (Please see the first page of this book for details on how to access this content.)

Overview of Problem-Solving Method

Problem-Solving Method (Figure 2.1 in text)
Problem-Solving Definitions (Table 2.1 in text)

Define D1: Situation and Scope

Project Consulting Agreement

Define D2: Stakeholders, Difficulties, and Problem Areas

Stakeholder Analysis Table
Problem Area Summary Table
Interview Guide

Define D3: Issue Statements and Problem Statement

Problem Area Summary Table

Study S1: Root Causes and Alternative Solutions

Stakeholder Analysis Table
Problem Area Summary Table

Study S2: Decision Criteria, Research, and Findings

Stakeholder Analysis Table
Problem Area Decision Criteria Table
Research Plan
Interview Guide

Study S3: Conclusions

Problem Area Decision Criteria Table

Act A1: Recommendations and Milestones

Problem Area Decision Criteria Table
Recommendations, Milestones, and Monitoring Measures
Key Milestones Gantt Chart

Act A2: Communication Strategy and Consensus Building

Stakeholder Analysis Table
Communication Plan
Example Executive Summary Outline
Final Presentation Strategy Checklist

Act A3: Implementation and Monitoring

Recommendations, Milestones, and Monitoring Measures

PART 1

THE MINDSET AND METHOD FOR PROBLEM-SOLVING

CHAPTER 1

THE PROBLEM IS NOT ALWAYS WHAT IT SEEMS

INTRODUCTION

Whenever I run into a problem I can't solve, I always make it bigger. I can never solve it by trying to make it smaller, but if I make it big enough, I begin to see the outlines of a solution.[1]

—*General Dwight D. Eisenhower*

In your career as a healthcare leader, you will be called upon every day to solve problems. Some problems will be big problems, others may seem like small ones. But even the problems that seem small and simple on the surface may have underlying components that, if not addressed, will prevent the seemingly simple problem from being resolved. How do you avoid making the problem smaller or simpler than it is, resulting in not solving the real problem? What does it mean to make the problem bigger, as General Dwight D. Eisenhower said? And, how big is big enough?

Do a web search on the words "problem-solving process," and almost without exception, the process descriptions returned in the search will state "define the problem" as an early step. But how do you define the problem? Ask a group of people to define the problem, and some will speculate about root causes, some will make assumptions that are their own opinions, some will ask for more information, some will jump to potential solutions, and some will mention a subset of symptoms. But none of these answers defines what the problem is. If there is not agreement on the definition of the problem, it will be difficult to arrive at an agreed upon solution to resolve it.

Our goal in writing *Applied Problem-Solving in Healthcare Management* is, first and foremost, to help you develop the discernment to recognize and define problems in a way that "makes the problem bigger" while simultaneously driving consensus on the problem definition. And once the problem has been defined, you will learn how to systematically study the problem to arrive at action-oriented recommendations that, when implemented, will resolve the problem as stated.

We do this by introducing you to the problem-solving method that has been taught in the University of Minnesota Master of Healthcare Administration (MHA) Program since its inception. The method, called the Minnesota MHA Method of Problem-Solving, has three phases—define, study, and act—each of which has a number of steps. For brevity's sake, we refer to it as "the Problem-Solving Method" in the remainder of this text. It is a disciplined, structured, and logical approach to solving problems that has been successful for young students, early careerists, and seasoned leaders.

As described later in this first chapter, simply following the steps by rote in the Problem-Solving Method will not ensure problem-solving success. Successful problem-solving requires that you develop a problem-solving mindset of a "never assume" attitude. This "never assume" attitude requires that you must be able to step outside of yourself and your view of the problem, you must actively listen to the stakeholders affected by the problem to understand it from their perspective, and you must avoid prematurely jumping to solutions that you think will fix the problem.

Learning how to develop a "never assume" mindset and how to apply each step of the method takes practice. Thus, in this first chapter we will introduce you to a student team eager to begin their consulting project, described in their case "The Spinal Frontier." If you are not a student, the case is still applicable, as this could very well be a consulting project or an internal project for a team in an organization. We start the case here to showcase how the first few project meetings relate to the title of this chapter—the problem is not always what it seems.

After describing the results of the students' initial meetings with their host organization, we describe how their experience is not uncommon as you try to unpack what the "real" problem is when working in organizations. We next describe in this chapter what is required of you to develop a "never assume" mindset as the prerequisite for applying the steps of the Problem-Solving Method. We then describe two types of intelligence—crystallized and fluid—to highlight that even with limited real-world experience, you can become an expert in solving healthcare problems using the systematic approach of the Problem-Solving Method. We end this first chapter with a description of the rest of the problem-solving text and how to use it to learn and apply the method.

CASE: THE SPINAL FRONTIER

The students were excited to start their consulting project during their last semester of study. They attended the first class session, where they learned who their team members would be and the organization in which they would be doing their project. The student team assigned to Prism Health System was especially excited about their project. As described in the summary provided to them by their consulting project faculty advisor, the project involved value-based care and care coordination for a chronic health condition in a health system that also owns and operates its own health plan. Exhibit 1.1 contains the written summary project description the students received during their initial consulting project class meeting.

After the students received their consulting project information from their faculty advisor, the student who agreed to be the project manager for the team scheduled a kick-off meeting at Prism Health System's headquarters with their organizational preceptors, Dr. LaTonya Waters and Mr. Anthony Hayden, the Musculoskeletal Clinical Service Line dyad leads. The dyad leaders also invited to the meeting Mr. Hayden's boss, the Prism

EXHIBIT 1.1

THE SPINAL FRONTIER CONSULTING PROJECT DESCRIPTION

Prism Health System Student Consulting Project

Organization Background: Prism Health System is located in a Midwestern state known for its progressive healthcare. It is a highly integrated system, both vertically and horizontally. Prism's delivery system consists of a large multispecialty group practice of 200+ physicians, a 300 bed community hospital, three critical access hospitals, and several satellite clinics and outpatient service sites. The system was formed 10 years ago through the merger of the Prism Medical Group and the former Westport Hospital. The system has strong financials, solid market share, top quartile quality scores, and an excellent community reputation.

Prism also owns and operates a health plan, which began 1 year after the merger. The health plan has also been successful. It has grown to 150,000 members, of which 90% are commercial members via employer contracts, and 10% are in its Medicare Advantage product that has a Five Star Rating. The Prism Health System executive team views the health plan as their window into the employer and consumer markets, especially from a cost and value perspective, and as part of Prism's very public commitment to the Triple Aim.

Two years ago, Prism Health System started a Musculoskeletal Clinical Service Line to coordinate program development across the system for its patients with spine problems, such as chronic neck and back pain. The service line is managed using a dyad partner model comprising a physician and an administrator. It is guided by a steering group comprising key clinicians and executives.

Consulting Project Deliverable: Prism Health System's cost of providing spine care is high compared to insurance industry local, regional, and national benchmarks. To reduce the costs of providing spine care while maintaining quality and patient outcomes, the Prism Musculoskeletal Clinical Service Line Dyad Leaders are planning to enter into a joint venture with MedSpine, a national company that specializes in low-cost, high-quality spine care. The project deliverable is to develop a plan to implement the joint venture.

Prism Organizational Preceptors: Musculoskeletal Service Line dyad leads: LaTonya Waters, MD, an orthopedic surgeon, and Anthony Hayden, MHA.

Health System Chief Operating Officer (COO), Charles Dressen, which was great exposure for the student team. The students learn the following during their meeting.

Anthony Hayden (Administrative Dyad): "It wasn't that long ago that I was in your shoes. I received my master's degree in health administration 5 years ago. After finishing my post-graduate fellowship here at Prism, I was hired as a member of Prism's Quality Improvement staff. After 3 years in that role, I was hired a little over a year ago into my current role as the administrative dyad partner for the Musculoskeletal Clinical Service Line. In addition to my service line director role, the Physical Therapy and Occupational Therapy Directors both report to me. I report to our Prism Health System COO, Charles Dressen, and I am happy he is able to join us today for this kick-off meeting."

Dr. LaTonya Waters (Clinical Dyad): "Prism Health System switched to a clinical service line organizational structure a couple of years ago to better coordinate care across the system for patients with chronic conditions. I was appointed as the clinician lead for the Musculoskeletal Clinical Service Line, and I work closely with my dyad administrative partner Anthony. The specialities in our Musculoskeletal Service Line include Orthopedics, Sports Medicine, and a nonsurgical program, Rheumatology. Each of these specialties also has a dyad leadership model. Our goal for the service line is to coordinate program development for spine care across our health system.

"We want to be recognized as the provider of choice by the community for spine care. We recently hired a new Spine Surgeon, Dr. Grant Norton, to build a spine surgery program, and that has been progressing well. We have a thriving orthopedics program that my immediate boss, Dr. Diwakar Patel, the Chair of Orthopedics, is very dedicated to and is proud of the teams performance."

"We have put a Musculoskeletal Clinical Service Line Steering Committee in place to provide input into decisions about the service line. The Steering Committee comprises our COO Charles, Dr. Norton, Nadeem Aziz—the CEO of Prism Health Plan, Sarah Wallace—the CFO of our main hospital, Dr. Patel, and of course, Anthony and me. Dr. Patel and I co-chair the Steering Committee. The Steering Committee meets quarterly, and although it doesn't have formal voting authority, it is very influential and we listen closely to the opinions expressed by everyone during our meetings. You will be presenting your recommendations about the joint venture plan to the Steering Committee, and we will invite other key members of the team who are impacted by the recommendations to your final presentation."

Anthony Hayden (Administrative Dyad): "I'd like to provide you with some background of how we got to this decision of a joint venture. I was at a meeting a couple of months ago with Nadeem Aziz, the Prism Health Plan CEO. During the meeting, he provided me with data and told me that the cost of providing spine care for Prism Health System patients is high compared to insurance industry local, regional, and national benchmarks, and is rising rapidly. He told me this is making it difficult to price the Prism Health Plan's products at a competitive premium rate.

"This was surprising to Dr. Waters and me, as our internal data, although incomplete, signaled that the service line efforts were tracking on point for revenue and utilization. Our internal physical therapy's volume had picked up alongside surgical volumes, and we have seen increased musculoskeletal imaging volumes."

"At that meeting, Nadeem strongly encouraged me to talk with MedSpine, a national company that specializes in spine care. MedSpine provides nonsurgical spine care at lower costs. The group, which was founded by an orthopedic surgeon and an exercise physiologist, is a provider of nonsurgical, intensive exercise- and strengthening-based care to patients with chronic neck and back pain. He had encouraged me to connect with MedSpine a number of months earlier, but I didn't have the time or see the need to connect until he told me about our costs of spine care being high compared to benchmarks."

Dr. LaTonya Waters (Clinical Dyad): "Anthony and I researched MedSpine, including reviewing peer-reviewed articles. The published studies report a more than 50% reduction in surgical procedures, major cost savings, and positive patient outcomes, as measured by Oswestry scores, when compared to patients who undergo spine surgery. We found their results to be convincing enough that we decided that we should meet with MedSpine."

Anthony Hayden (Administrative Dyad): "I recently met with MedSpine. Shortly thereafter, the MedSpine leadership team sent us an initial proposal to form a joint venture with them to own and operate a MedSpine program at Prism Health System. Although I have had heard pushback from some folks in the hospital, a joint venture with MedSpine is going to position us well given our health system's commitment to the Triple Aim."

Charles Dressen (COO): "Our initial vetting of the MedSpine proposal is that it looks good. It appears profitable, it is clinically efficient with high quality providers, the Health Plan sees value in the organization, and our attorney says the contract looks good. I find it all very promising.

"It is important that we get moving on this. A strategic wrinkle in the situation is that Nadeem informed us that they will be establishing a Spine Center of Distinction Program that is based on outcomes and costs, and they would like to pilot bundled payments with the 'right partner.' Nadeem made a comment to me that our services lines, including our Musculoskeletal Service line, 'need to start acting like real service lines in today's world of value-based care' if we want to be considered as the 'right partner.' So, time is of the essence, and we need to get a plan in place for moving forward on this joint venture."

The students were provided with names and contact information for a number of key stakeholders with whom they should meet as they work on their project, and discussed how to best keep their preceptors updated on their progress.

The student team was able to set up three back-to-back meetings the following Monday morning with three stakeholders on their list: Dr. Grant Norton—the recently hired spine surgeon, Sarah Wallace—the hospital CFO, and Andrea Meyer—the Director of Physical Therapy. Here is some of what they heard in these meetings.

Dr. Grant Norton (Spine Surgeon): "I heard second-hand from Sarah Wallace about the proposed joint venture. Frankly, I was surprised, as this was the first I'd heard about it. A joint venture has never been discussed at our Steering Committee meetings. I was brought here to build a spine surgery program, and all indications are that I am doing it very successfully. I am not convinced this nonsurgical approach is good for patients. Why haven't I been involved in these discussions? I called Anthony to let him know my feelings, but I guess they have decided to move forward anyway."

Andrea Meyer (Director of Physical Therapy): "Why would we bring someone from the outside to do this? I told Anthony that I think this is a bad idea for at least two reasons. First, the joint venture will take volume from my department and I will have to lay off staff. Second, the orthopedic surgeons have never wanted to get involved in a program like this. We don't even have any real protocols for managing patients with chronic neck and back pain. Why haven't I been involved in any of the discussions about this?"

Sarah Wallace (Hospital CFO): "I told Anthony that the MedSpine joint venture will reduce spine surgery and imaging volume, which will hurt the hospital's revenue and operating margin. It might save the Prism Health Plan money, but it will hurt the hospital, the current physical therapy department and surgeons. I also don't understand why the Health Plan should be dictating what clinical care we should be offering in our service lines. We should be deciding that.

"I know there are strong opinions in our organization about this proposed joint venture. There are many of us that are concerned that we are jumping to a terrible solution. I think right now this is too political to be appropriate for a student project. Let's pause this project for now until I can talk with Dr. Waters, Anthony, and the rest of our Steering Committee, and we'll get back to you."

NOW WHAT?

Well, that put a damper on the student team's enthusiasm for the project, and some team members were worried that this project may be canceled. The four team members, Tatiana, Patrick, Gabriella, and Jayden, spent the rest of Monday afternoon discussing and sometimes arguing among themselves about what is going on at Prism Health System and what to do next.

Tatiana, the team member with a year of clinical experience as a medical assistant for a spine surgeon, agreed with the physical therapist and hospital CFO:

Nonsurgical treatment of neck and back pain does not work, and surgery is almost always eventually needed for chronic back pain. Since hospitals make money on surgery and pay the surgeons' salaries, the joint venture would be devastating for the hospital's financial position.

Patrick majored in psychology as an undergraduate and worked for 2 years in the human resources department prior to starting his master's degree. He was attuned to watching people's facial expressions and body language.

Did you see how Charles, the COO raised his eyebrows and Dr. Waters looked at her phone when Anthony mentioned that some folks at the hospital aren't on board with the joint venture? I am wondering if our site sponsors are not recognizing the full extent of their colleagues' concerns. And, why did they send us out to meet with people that are against a joint venture without warning us ahead of time? Do they even know what the others believe? It would seem like at least the system COO would know that the hospital CFO is not on board. Are we going to have to convince the CFO to go forward with the joint venture—is that really the project? It seems like we are being set up for failure.

Gabriella was quiet during most of the meeting and noncommittal about whether the joint venture was or wasn't a good idea. She instead tied what they were seeing at Prism back to what they had learned from a CEO who was a recent guest speaker in their integrated delivery systems class.

Remember what our guest speaker said last week in class? The health plan's costs are the delivery system's revenues. There is bound to be a conflict if, on the one hand, they are trying to compete in a value-based Triple Aim world, but on the other hand, they are rewarding their delivery system leaders for revenue production. It's that canoe story. The health system has to keep one foot on the dock to succeed in the current environment and have one foot in the canoe to move to the new value-based environment. They need to find the right balance to know when to push off from the dock and put both feet in the canoe. Maybe our project should be more about the various options for the service line to reduce costs and improve quality, and less about the MedSpine joint venture specifically.

Jayden, who worked as a project manager for an engineering firm prior to starting his master's studies, sided with Anthony and Charles's position.

Look, if the joint venture isn't implemented, Prism's own health plan is going to choose a different strategic partner for their Spine Center of Distinction Program. The CFO and other people who are opposed to the joint venture need to realize that it's a new world out there. Anthony, Charles, and Dr. Waters need to just tell people this is how it's going to be and get on with it. We need to tell our faculty advisor that we should move ahead with the project to show that the MedSpine joint venture is the best option, as described to us by our preceptors, and to ask our faculty advisor to call Anthony to reaffirm our project deliverable.

The team argued to an impasse and felt they had wasted the last 4 hours spinning their wheels and getting frustrated that their teammates had differing views of the problem. They emailed their faculty advisor saying they needed to meet with her as soon as possible because it looks like they may need a different project and/or a meeting to figure this out with the organization.

How might using the Problem-Solving Method have helped the students in these first few days of their consulting project?

The Musculoskeletal Clinical Service Line leaders and the Prism Health System COO clearly think the MedSpine joint venture is a strategic imperative, while the hospital CFO, the spine surgeon, and the physical therapy director disagree. If the students had learned and practiced the Problem-Solving Method prior to their meetings, they could have moved the project forward in these early stages with less angst and spinning of their wheels. They might have asked some probing questions in their kickoff meeting to understand the logic behind how the service line leadership dyad came to the joint venture decision. They would have realized that the hospital CFO and others are bringing their own perspectives that need further exploration. Their follow-up meeting with their faculty advisor would have been more proactively focused on how the project scope should be renegotiated with Prism Health System to explore other options beyond the MedSpine joint venture for achieving the goals of the service line given the lack of agreement in the organization around the best course of action. And they would have recognized the need for thoroughly understanding all of the key stakeholders' viewpoints as they engage in their project.

On the faculty side, if they had experience with the Problem-Solving Method, the advisor would have facilitated the development of the project deliverable with the organization such that there was a problem to be solved, not just a solution to be implemented. This helps avoid a Type III error, which we describe in the following paragraph. Student consulting projects should require that all three phases of the Problem-Solving Method—Define, Study, and Act—need to be explored by the student team. Generally, student projects with a sole deliverable of how to implement a pre-determined solution from the organization should be avoided.

TYPE III ERROR

The student team encountered a common situation—a Type III error. You hopefully remember the terms Type I error and Type II error from your statistics classes. A Type I error is rejecting the null hypothesis when you shouldn't. A Type II error is not rejecting the null hypothesis when you should. But you probably didn't discuss a Type III error—*"solving the wrong problem"*[2(p383)] or *"solving the trivial problem rather than the most important problem given the resources and needs of the organization."*[3]

What the students are experiencing at Prism Health Care is what many professionals, at all levels, experience with their organizations and teams. In The Spinal Frontier case, perhaps the Musculoskeletal Service Line dyad leaders and the Prism Health System COO investigated a range of alternative solutions, and a joint venture with MedSpine was determined to be the best course of action for Prism Health System. At this point, the students do not know if other alternatives were investigated and rejected.

And, that does not negate the other interrelated problems that the students uncovered in the conversations they have had with three other stakeholders—people feeling like their views are being ignored, people feeling afraid that their or their department's performance will suffer, people feeling angry, potential for financial losses to the hospital, people disagreeing about the joint venture being the best course of action. These problems all need to be addressed to successfully move the organization forward.

If you have ever been in a meeting where the conversation gets stuck because people are arguing about what the "right" solution is, you are likely experiencing an example of a Type III error. Different people in the meeting actually have different unstated views about what the problem is. If there is not agreement on the facts of what the problem is, there certainly will not be agreement about the best solution on how to resolve it. And, when people provide their viewpoints of what the problem is, they will often frame it in terms of a solution:

> "We need to open another operating room so surgeons can get timely access on the schedule."

> "If administration wants us to finish by the end of the shift, we need more nursing staff."

> "We need physicians to abide by the vacation policy because they are canceling clinics."

> "Telemedicine will fix our access issues."

> "We need to hire a new physician to ensure the sustainability of the division."

> "If the nurses would just push the button in the bed tracking system, we would know that the bed is available for cleaning."

> "Our hospital is always running at bed capacity, we need to add a new bed tower."

> "We need to develop a joint venture with MedSpine to reduce our cost of spine care while still maintaining quality and outcomes of care."

The problem as defined for the students by the Prism Health System Musculoskeletal Clinical Service Line leaders was to develop an implementation plan for a joint venture with MedSpine (a solution). But, this is only one possible solution (joint venture) to achieve a goal (reduce our cost of spine care while maintaining quality and outcomes). The hospital CFO does not agree with that definition of the problem. And she identified a different goal—avoid harming the finances of the hospital. The physical therapist had an additional goal—do not do anything that results in her having to lay off staff. The spine surgeon was confused—he has been successful in generating surgical and imaging volume, and now they want just the opposite. The problem definition has implicitly devolved into a dichotomy—should a joint venture with MedSpine be undertaken, or shouldn't it?

So what can be done to resolve these conversations that get "stuck"? Solving the right problem requires defining the problem correctly. The challenge of problem solving is not to determine who is right and who is wrong, and then implement the solution of the person who is right. The purpose is to accurately define what the problem is and to arrive at a best acceptable and implementable solution that fixes the problem and its root causes, and that moves the organization forward towards its goals and vision for the future. As you will see in Chapter 2, the problem definition approach of the Problem-Solving Method taught in this text is to learn how to articulate the key questions that need to be answered to solve the problem.

How can you define the problem "correctly"? Many people in the organization will have a variety of perceptions and viewpoints about the problem, its root causes, their preferred alternative solutions, and their goals for seeing their view of the problem resolved.

A good problem solver will talk to as many people as practical and possible in the time frame available to gain these multiple perspectives. All of them will have insights, and all will likely have varying perspectives.

The analogy is the story of the six blind men describing an elephant they are touching for the first time.[4] Each of the men touches a different part of the elephant – the side, the trunk, the tail, the leg, the tusk, and the ear. And then each of them describes the elephant based on the part of the elephant touched. They are all partly right, but also partly wrong because they assume that their experience is a complete description of an elephant. It is only in synthesizing their viewpoints that a complete picture emerges of what an elephant looks like.

Leaders who are effective problem solvers excel at asking the right questions of the right people and analyzing, synthesizing, and integrating those views, along with other research, data, and fact-finding, to determine what the problem actually is and how it might best be resolved.

PROBLEMS ARE "MESSES"

> Managers are not confronted with problems that are independent of each other, but with dynamic situations that consist of complex systems of changing problems that interact with each other. I call such situations messes. Problems are abstractions extracted from messes by analysis....Managers do not solve problems; they manage messes.[5]
>
> —Russell Ackoff (1979, pp. 99–100)

The challenge is that rarely is there just one stand-alone problem that can be identified and resolved. Instead, Russell Ackoff, a famous organizational systems theorist, described organizational problems as being interconnected and interdependent. A problem cannot be solved in isolation of the other surrounding problems in which it is embedded. Instead, interrelated problems must be solved and resolved systematically. Problems are complex, and they are "messy."

The challenge for organizational leaders is that there is usually limited time to sit back and admire a problem in all of its messy interrelatedness. At some point, a decision about a preferred course of action must be made and implemented, often with very limited information and time. But it is possible to develop the capability to quickly assess and study problem interrelatedness when solving "the mess" that is the problem.

It is important that the solution to today's problem is not the root cause of tomorrow's problem. The Problem-Solving Method taught in this text will help keep you from jumping to solutions that lead to Type III errors, and will help you develop a way of thinking that facilitates an almost subconscious thought process that enables you to quickly identify the interrelated components of messy problems.

NEVER ASSUME

Why are problem definitions with embedded solutions "problematic"? Solution-based problem definitions assume a solution without clearly identifying what the problem is that needs fixing. Such statements assume that the correct single root cause has been identified in their solution—lack of a resource or incompetent colleagues, for example. The statements assume their single solution will fix what may be a messy problem with interrelated components. The problem solver might assume they know the motives of colleagues and place blame. And the problem solver often assumes the problem lies with someone else, not themselves.

When gathering, analyzing, synthesizing, and integrating a variety of viewpoints, data, and observations to define and solve a problem, it is important to maintain a "never assume" attitude. Broadly speaking, to never assume is to avoid rushing to judgment. A never assume attitude has three components. First, understand yourself. Second, understand your stakeholders. Third, develop the discipline of engaging in cycles of divergent and convergent thinking. In the Problem-Solving Method, you need to engage in divergent thinking to "make the problem bigger" before converging to a problem definition. And you need to engage in a second cycle of divergent thinking when brainstorming and studying a range of possible root causes and potential alternative solutions before converging on a recommended course of action.

■ UNDERSTAND YOURSELF

To know that we know what we know, and to know that we do not know what we do not know, that is true knowledge.[6]

—*Nicolaus Copernicus*

What gets us into trouble is not what we don't know. It's what we know for sure that just ain't so.[7]

—*Mark Twain*

A strength of The Spinal Frontier student project team is that each of them brings diverse knowledge to the team. However, their past experiences may be creating bias in their views of the problem. Based on her previous clinical experience, Tatiana assumes that the nonsurgical MedSpine treatment approach is not effective. Patrick assumes what Charles Dressen was thinking based on his raising an eyebrow, and he assumes that Anthony and Dr. Waters are not listening to their colleagues. Gabriella assumes this is a classic conflict seen in health systems with a health plan, and Jayden assumes that those not supporting the joint venture just don't understand the value-based imperative of today's healthcare environment.

Similar assumptions can also be seen in the Prism Health System actors. The CFO assumes the hospital will lose money, and the physical therapy director assumes that staff will need to be laid off with the joint venture. Conversely, the Prism Health System COO and Service Line leadership dyad, and the health plan CEO, assume that the MedSpine joint venture is needed to stay competitive as a health system.

To be an effective, logical problem solver, you need a "never assume" attitude. This requires that you recognize your own values, experiences, and world-view, and question how they might be shaping subconscious assumptions you may have about the problem.

You need to develop the capability to factually identify what you know about the problem, and what you know you don't know about the problem. But most importantly, you need to recognize that what you think you know for sure might not be true—never assume.

If you have a particular set of values, you need to be clear about what they are and determine if they may cloud your ability to define the problem in an impartial way. If there is a coworker you do not get along with, you need to ensure that you don't infer intentions in their behavior that are not accurate or question their motives. If you are working in an organization and the problem is affecting you or those who report to you, then you need to recognize that you may be part of the problem. If there is something about the problem that is making you angry, you need to acknowledge the anger and be able to step outside of it. If you have a bias toward a particular solution, you need to ensure you do not ignore other possible solutions. If you focus on your preferred solution, and only seek out evidence that supports your preferred solution, then you are in danger of confirmation bias.[8] This is defined as the tendency to interpret new evidence as confirming your existing beliefs or theories, while ignoring contrary evidence that could refute them.

A "never assume" attitude requires that in any situation in which you are engaged in problem-solving, you step outside of yourself, as if you are an impartial external consultant viewing the problem, and also ask yourself if you are part of the problem. *Never assume that you are not part of the problem.* Thus, the ability to be a "never assume" problem solver requires self-awareness (accurate self-perception of the impact of your emotions on your behaviors and actions) and self-regulation (the ability to control your emotions, desires, and behaviors).[9]

The need to "never assume" does not decrease as you gain experience in problem-solving. In fact, you may need to be more attentive to a "never assume" attitude as you progress in your career. Daniel Kahneman, a Nobel Prize winning psychologist and economist, and his colleague, Amos Tversky, a cognitive and mathematical psychologist, spent their careers studying why people make suboptimal decisions. Their joint research on judgment and decision-making identified heuristics and biases that can affect our decisions. For example, as you gain experience, you may judge a solution to be preferred because of a bias called availability bias—you remember it as a solution that has worked before, and you will judge it as having a high probability of being successful in this situation as it is easily retrieved from your memory.[10]

As your career progresses, relying on your experiences when solving organizational problems can be helpful. But experience might also cause you to prematurely decide on a course of action based on the memories of your experiences. This might lull you into limiting your efforts in being thorough in defining the interrelated mess that is the problem because you "remember this problem from before." Or, you remember a solution that worked recently or frequently, rather than searching for a range of possible alternative solutions that would result in a novel solution that is better than before. Never assume.

■ UNDERSTAND YOUR STAKEHOLDERS

A stakeholder is a person, group of people, unit, department, organization, or other entity, either internal or external, that is affected by the problem in some way. Some stakeholders may be more directly impacted by the problem, while others may be more indirectly affected. When solving a problem, it is important to identify the stakeholders affected by the situation and talk to them to gather their perceptions, perspectives, and feelings about the situation.

Your goal in talking with them is to understand the situation and how it affects them as they perceive it. You are there to observe, listen, and learn to develop that understanding, not to tell them they are wrong or challenge or pass judgment on their viewpoint. You do not question their motives, even if they are exhibiting behaviors that you do not understand. Your "never assume" attitude requires that you ask thoughtful, probing, respectful questions to gather the perspectives, perceptions, and feelings of key stakeholders to the problem in a systematic and nonjudgmental way to gain insights into the problem and how it might be resolved.

Truly listening to stakeholders doesn't mean they will get the solutions they prefer. But it provides you as the problem solver with an understanding of the criteria that the different stakeholders value if the problem is to be successfully resolved in their eyes. As you work through alternative solutions, some of which were generated by your stakeholders, and others which were identified through your research in studying the problem, you will need to judge the relative merits of possible alternative solutions against these criteria. The Problem-Solving Method you will learn in this text requires a systematic stakeholder analysis.

■ DIVERGENT AND CONVERGENT THINKING

A way to recognize and step out of your own world view and potential bias is to work through cycles of divergent and convergent thinking. Divergent thinking involves generating as many ideas as possible without judging at the time whether they are "good" or "bad" ideas. In problem-solving, divergent thinking involves generating as many ideas as possible about what the problem is, what its root causes might be, and what alternative solutions might eliminate those root causes.

This is why a thorough stakeholder analysis is so important—it helps generate a variety of ideas that should be investigated. Of course, other methods are also needed to engage in divergent thinking in problem-solving, such as data analysis, direct observation, reading published literature related to the problem, and brainstorming.

Divergent thinking in problem-solving is important because what appears on the surface to be a simple problem may have many layers of complexity to it. And seldom will a problem be solved with one single-pronged solution. If the definition of the problem has a solution embedded in it, it prevents resolving the real underlying root causes of the problem and prematurely cuts off considering other solutions. The first solution that comes to mind, the least expensive one, the fastest one to implement, or the one that another organization has implemented, might not be the best solution in this particular situation.

Divergent thinking helps you avoid prematurely jumping to simplistic views of the problem and solutions that don't address its root causes. A "never assume" attitude during divergent thinking means that you keep your mind open to all possible ideas, and do not ignore or eliminate them until you have systematically evaluated them. You do not prematurely jump to rash conclusions or decisions.

The logical process of systematically analyzing the ideas generated during divergent thinking is called "convergent thinking." In convergent thinking, you study, analyze, synthesize and integrate the ideas generated during divergent thinking to arrive at a summary that accurately captures its results. In the Problem-Solving Method, convergent thinking leads to a definition of the problem, its identified actual root causes, and solutions that should be implemented to eliminate the root causes.

The Problem-Solving Method taught in this text takes you through two waves of divergent and convergent thinking, as shown in Figure 1.1. These two divergent–convergent waves of thinking are analogous to what has been coined as the "Double Diamond" in Design Thinking.[11]

The first wave of divergent and convergent thinking occurs in the Define phase. In this phase, you engage in divergent thinking as you explore the situation to identify the inter-related complexities of the problem. You then engage in convergent thinking to define the problem, arriving at a problem statement and a vision for the future if the problem is successfully resolved.

The second wave of divergent thinking occurs in the Study phase. In this phase, divergent thinking is used to brainstorm possible root causes of the problem and potential alternative solutions to eliminate them. Through conducting research and analysis in the Study phase, you collect facts that enable you to converge on a set of conclusions

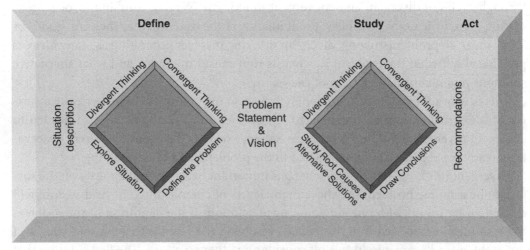

FIGURE 1.1 The Problem-Solving Method's "Double Diamond" waves of divergent–convergent thinking.

about the preferred course of action. This results in a set of recommendations that are implemented in the last phase of the Problem-Solving Method—the Act phase. There are multiple steps in each of these phases that will be described in detail in Chapter 2.

BECOMING AN EXPERT PROBLEM SOLVER

Problem-solving and decision-making form the basis of most leadership activities. A healthcare leader's potential for success depends heavily on their ability to sort out and solve problems effectively. Leaders are constantly confronted with multiple interrelated problems in the organization that need attention, and the interrelatedness means the problems cannot be solved in isolation of each other. Therefore, effective leaders need to learn and internalize a well-developed approach to problem-solving that enables them to quickly sort out what the problem is, what the goals of the problem-solving process are, what parts of the process require their direct attention, which parts should be delegated to others, and ensuring that solutions that actually fix the problem are successfully implemented and evaluated to move the organization forward.

From what you have read so far, you may be thinking it will take you years of experience to become an expert in solving problems. After all, there are many professionals in the field who have many more years of experience than you. Nothing could be further from the truth. Think about the student team in The Spinal Frontier case and the situation they face. The Prism Health System leadership team and clinicians are very smart people with years of experience. Yet they are in a predicament of their own making and it is causing disagreement. The student team can help them through this predicament by bringing a disciplined approach to problem-solving.

A theory of intelligence developed by the psychologist Raymond Cattell posits that there are two types of intelligence—crystallized and fluid.[12,13] Crystallized intelligence is the ability to use knowledge gained through past experience and this increases with age. As you work in the healthcare field, you will gain contextual knowledge about the industry and how it works, and thus your crystallized intelligence will develop.

In contrast, fluid intelligence does not require prior experience or knowledge about the situation. Fluid intelligence is the ability to use logic and reasoning to solve problems in novel situations. The theory posits that fluid intelligence is greater in younger people, and diminishes with age.

Therefore, even with limited healthcare experience, students and early careerists can develop their fluid intelligence through learning a structured, logical process to solve problems for which they have little real-world crystallized intelligence. And, in the process of using the Problem-Solving Method, you will develop your crystallized intelligence about the healthcare system and how it works.

Healthcare leaders will tell you that almost every day they face novel problems for which they could never have been taught a "right" answer. Thus, even with years of crystallized intelligence, leaders frequently face new situations that require fluid intelligence. Every day brings new situations, and a key role of the leader is to help the organization sort out and solve these problems efficiently and effectively.

Sometimes the problem manifests itself as a conversation in the hallway, and the leader can help facilitate its resolution in a matter of minutes. Sometimes the problem requires months of study by a project team to whom the leader has delegated responsibility for defining and studying the problem to arrive at a set of recommendations. Whether the problem-solving process takes 3 minutes in the hallway or 3 months of meetings, the leader has to have an intuitive "never assume" mindset that is second nature when approaching and solving the problem, and model this mindset for others in the organization.

As is true for developing any skill, it takes practice to master becoming a "never assume" problem solver. You have to practice to learn how to ride a bike. You have to practice to learn how to play the piano. You have to practice to learn how to play hockey. You have to practice to learn how to solve problems. Most programs in health administration require students to practice problem-solving by completing a consulting project or summer internship to solve a real-world problem in an organization. And there are many case-based courses and student case competitions that provide opportunities to solve simulated healthcare industry problems. After graduating, you will continue to hone your problem-solving expertise, helping you develop leadership competencies to successfully lead as you progress in your career.

This text provides the Problem-Solving Method and a set of tools and practice activities to help you develop the skills to become a successful "never assume" problem solver. For young students and early careerists, the Problem-Solving Method provides a structured framework, tools, and mindset to successfully engage in real-world projects early in your studies or career, even when you have limited experience or expertise with a given topic. The Problem-Solving Method helps you develop a problem-solving discipline to never assume, to not jump to solutions, to listen to stakeholders, to understand the context of the problem, to engage in productive cycles of divergent and convergent thinking, to arrive at a comprehensive problem definition, to identify root causes of the problem and not just its symptoms, to develop skills to research the problem, its root causes, and solutions, and to focus on strategies for gaining stakeholder acceptance of recommended solutions.

Experienced leaders who use the Problem-Solving Method find that with practice, the steps and principles come naturally without consciously thinking about them. It becomes intuitive, and they are able to use the Problem-Solving Method to quickly synthesize and integrate large volumes of information from inside and outside the organization. They will rarely, if ever, write out the steps. And they may not complete all the steps every time a problem arises. It is the mindset that helps them ask the key questions of themselves and their stakeholders that are needed to discern what the problem is and to take appropriate actions that move their organizations toward its vision and goals while solving the problem at hand. They model the "never assume" leadership behavior of the Problem-Solving Method as part of their responsibilities that serves as a role model and values for others in the organization.

Practicing the "never assume" principles is as important as mastering the steps of the Problem-Solving Method. Mindlessly working through the steps and using the associated tools and templates will not guarantee problem-solving success. The "never assume" principle requires that you be objective, factual, and logical. You need to recognize and set aside your personal biases and preconceived notions. You need to acknowledge to yourself and others if you bring a priori beliefs, values, or assumptions to the problem, and not let them affect your objectivity. You need to control your negative emotions and any over-excitement. You need to avoid making assumptions about others' motives based on their behavior. You need to look inside yourself and ask if you are part of the problem. You need to avoid rushing to judgment. You need to step outside of the situation you are facing, as if you are an outside consultant looking in at the situation.

And another "never assume" principle is to truly listen to the stakeholders affected by the problem to understand their perspectives, perceptions, and feelings. You need to demonstrate compassion and empathy when working with stakeholders. Kaissi (2018) cites Tan (2010, p. 199) in describing the three components of compassion: I understand you (a cognitive component), I feel for you (an affective component), and I want to help you (a motivational component).[14,15] Empathy involves taking stakeholders' emotions into account as one aspect to consider when solving the problem.[16]

USING THE PROBLEM-SOLVING TEXT

Applied Problem-Solving in Healthcare Management is organized into four parts. Part I of the text comprises four chapters. It is designed to be a self-contained description of the Problem-Solving Method. Chapter 1 has provided you with the prerequisite knowledge you need to develop the mindset of a "never assume" problem solver.

Chapter 2 provides a detailed description of the Problem-Solving Method. The method is comprised of three phases—Define, Study, and Act. Each of these phases has three steps, and each of these steps, in turn, has several substeps. Definitions that are specific to the Problem-Solving Method are also provided. There is a lot to digest in Chapter 2, as it describes the "what" of each step of the Problem-Solving Method. As you gain experience in using the Problem-Solving Method, Chapter 2 will be useful as your reference guide when you need a refresher of what is entailed in any given step.

Chapters 3 and 4 provide information that you may want to wait to read until after you have worked through practicing the Problem-Solving Method in Parts II, III, and IV of the text. Chapter 3 compares and contrasts the Problem-Solving Method with two other frequently used problem-solving methods in healthcare today—Lean and Design Thinking—and describes how the Problem-Solving Method is complementary to, and not competing with, these other methods. The last chapter of Part I, Chapter 4, provides you with an overview of the leadership competencies you develop through learning and applying the Problem-Solving Method.

Parts II, III, and IV of the text are the "how-to" chapters for you to practice and apply the Problem-Solving Method. Part II covers the Define phase (Chapters 5 through 8), Part III covers the Study phase (Chapters 9 through 12), and Part IV covers the Act phase (Chapters 13 through 16). Each of the nine steps of the Problem-Solving Method has its own "how-to" chapter. Thus, there are three "how-to" chapters per part, since each phase of the Problem Solving Method has three steps. Each of these chapters provides a brief summary description of the substeps in each step, tips and tools for how to carry out the substeps, and activities to practice what you have learned. The Spinal Frontier case in Chapter 1 will serve as the case to which you will apply the activities. As you work through these chapters, you should refer back to Chapter 2 as a reference for more detail on each step and substep.

A fourth chapter in each part provides a key with answers and example responses for each of the activities in its "how-to" chapters. Many of the activities do not have a right or wrong answer. In these situations, the activity key provides detailed suggestions for how you might craft the answer for a given activity.

Give yourself plenty of time to work through these "how-to" chapters of the text. These chapters cannot and should not be completed in a single afternoon, for example. You need to think about and practice the activities in each of the Problem-Solving Method steps to learn and master them. You should write out your answers to the activities. As you complete each chapter in Parts II through IV of the text, you will be practicing its corresponding step of the Problem-Solving Method. Thus, for each chapter you will complete a substep of the method. The answers you develop for that chapter will be built upon as you tackle the next substep of the Problem-Solving Method in the next chapter. Thus, your work in each chapter builds cumulatively. When you have completed all of the steps, you will have solved the problem using the Problem-Solving Method.

Finally, Part V of the text provides a variety of cases for additional practice in using the Problem-Solving Method. These cases are organized into chapters based on broadly defined topics. Chapter 17 provides cases that focus on operations and quality, Chapter 18 provides cases that have a strategic focus, Chapter 19 provides cases that focus on population health, and Chapter 20 provides cases focused on long-term care. When practicing the method, you should write out each step. Circle back to Chapter 2 and the "how-to" chapters to guide your work. This will help you internalize the Problem-Solving Method, such that it simply becomes the way you think about and approach solving problems.

Remember, learning to apply the Problem-Solving Method is like learning any other skill. You have to practice. Practice on your own, practice with a friend, practice with a team. It takes time and practice to train your brain to make applying the steps and substeps of the Problem-Solving Method become part of your automatic thought process. As you engage in real-world consulting or internship, residency, or fellowship projects, come back to the Chapter 2 description of the Problem-Solving Method and each "how-to" chapter to reinforce your learning the method through real-world application.

REFERENCES

1. Lucco J. *The Eisenhower principle applied to business strategy management*. [Blog post]. 2019. https://www.clearpointstrategy.com/eisenhower-principle-and-business-strategy-management
2. Mitroff II, Featheringham TR. On systematic problem-solving and the error of the third kind. *Behav Sci*. 1974;19(6):383–393. doi:10.1002/bs.3830190605

3. Kilmann RH. Problem management: a behavioral science approach. In: Zaltman G, ed. *Management Principles for Nonprofit Agencies and Organizations*. New York, NY: American Management Association; 1979:213–255. https://kilmanndiagnostics.com/problem-management-a-behavioral-science-approach

4. Peace Corps. *The blind men and the elephant*. 2019. https://www.peacecorps.gov/educators/resources/story-blind-men-and-elephant

5. Ackoff RL. The future of operational research is past. *J Oper Res Soc*. 1979;30(2):93–104. doi:10.1057/jors.1979.22

6. BrainyQuote. 2019. https://www.brainyquote.com/quotes/nicolaus_copernicus_127510

7. Gurteen, D. *On what gets you into trouble by Mark Twain*. 2019. http://www.gurteen.com/gurteen/gurteen.nsf/id/what-gets-you-into-trouble

8. MacLean CL, Dror IE. A primer on the psychology of cognitive bias. In: Robertson CT, Kesselheim AS, eds. *Blinding as a solution to bias: Strengthening biomedical science, forensic science, and law*. New York, NY: Elsevier; 2016.

9. Chappelear J. Self-awareness and self-regulation: Core skills in effective leaders [online article]. *The Business Journals*. 2017. https://www.bizjournals.com/bizjournals/how-to/growth-strategies/2017/02/self-awareness-and-self-regulation-core-skills-in.html

10. Tversky A, Kahneman D. Availability: A heuristic for judging frequency and probability. *Cogn Psychol*. 1973;5(2):207–232. doi:10.1016/0010-0285(73)90033-9

11. Design Council. *What is the framework for innovation? Design Council's evolved Double Diamond*. 2019. https://www.designcouncil.org.uk/news-opinion/what-framework-innovation-design-councils-evolved-double-diamond

12. Horn JL, Cattell RB. Refinement and test of the theory of fluid and crystallized general intelligences. *J Educ Psychol*. 1966;57:253–270. doi:10.1037/h0023816

13. Horn JL, Cattell RB. Age differences in fluid and crystallized intelligence. *Acta Psychol*. 1967;26:107–129. doi:10.1016/0001-6918(67)90011-x

14. Kaissi A. *Intangibles: The unexpected traits of high-performing healthcare leaders*. Chicago, IL: Health Administration Press; 2018:74.

15. Tan C. *Search inside yourself: the unexpected path to achieving success, happiness (and world peace)*. New York, NY: HarperOne; 2010.

16. Goleman D. What makes a leader? *Harv Bus Rev*. 2004;82(1):82–91.

CHAPTER 2

THE PROBLEM-SOLVING METHOD

INTRODUCTION

As you scan through this chapter, you are likely excited to learn the Problem-Solving Method and at the same time may be thinking that it looks long and complicated, with all of the steps and substeps. And you may be wondering how healthcare leaders actually use the Problem-Solving Method as they carry out their responsibilities every day. We understand these thoughts and have been there ourselves when learning the Method. So, how does using the Problem-Solving Method ever become second nature to your thought process?

Think back to when you learned a new skill, like riding a bike. There were all those steps to remember—how to push off with one foot to get started, how to start gliding so you do not wobble, how to pedal, how to look straight ahead and not at your front wheel, how to balance, how to steer without running into a tree, how to brake without falling over. It was difficult because there were so many things you had to consciously think about, and you probably wobbled and fell often. But practice makes perfect, and then, one day, you realized that riding a bike had become automatic—the steps had become coordinated, seamless, and internalized, and you could ride a bike without thinking about it.

It is the same with learning the discipline of solving problems using the Problem-Solving Method. It takes practice to internalize the steps and terminology so that it becomes the way you automatically think. But once you have internalized them, you will hear a conversation, and automatically listen for *difficulties* to group into *problem areas* in your head. You will be able to quickly identify the *key issue* in each *problem area*. And you will *not* automatically jump to solutions. You will be able to do all this without having to think about it because it is just the way you think. The terms difficulties, problem areas, and issue statements are terms that have very specific meanings in the Problem-Solving Method. You have to learn what they mean and why they are important.

We have written Chapter 2 to serve as a reference guide—the one-stop location for the "what" of each step and substep of the Problem-Solving Method. It defines the terms specific to the Problem-Solving Method, and shows and describes all of the steps and substeps of each phase—step by step by step. As you practice and master the Problem-Solving Method, you will be able to come back to Chapter 2 to look up the details of each step and substep.

At the end of Chapter 2, we also provide a brief description of how the Problem-Solving Method is used in everyday problem-solving.

To learn the Problem-Solving Method, we recommend that you first just skim Chapter 2 to get an overall understanding of it. Do not try to memorize the Problem-Solving Method or worry if there is something that is not clear upon your initial reading. Then, after reading through this chapter, you should set aside time on a regular basis to practice the Problem-Solving Method by working through the chapters in Parts II, III, and IV of the text.

Parts II, III, and IV provide tools, tips, and activities for you to practice the Method so that you can learn it. Part II covers the Define phase, Part III covers the Study phase, and Part IV covers the Act phase. The chapters in Parts II, III, and IV are the "how-to" chapters, one chapter per step. As you work your way through those chapters, you should flip back to Chapter 2 to review the "what" and then work on the substep in its corresponding "how-to" chapter. Each of the "how-to" chapters builds on the previous one, so they should be completed sequentially. The activities in the "how-to" chapters require that you write out each activity. As you gain experience, you will rarely write out your problem-solving work—you will be able to do it in your head.

It should be noted that problem-solving does not mean that something must be "wrong" to use the Problem-Solving Method. Rather, the method is a process by which you can review any existing system or situation and determine if there is a more ideal future. If there is, or there is a desire or requirement to do an assessment or review, then the Problem-Solving Method serves as the reasoning "processor" for developing alternatives to the status quo of "doing nothing." And, in some situations, you may find that "doing nothing" is the preferred alternative at a given point in time.

As described in Chapter 1, successful problem-solving requires more than just completing each step of the Problem-Solving Method. It also requires the "never assume" mindset. This mindset includes understanding yourself, understanding your stakeholders, and engaging in divergent thinking to avoid prematurely jumping to solutions.

Understanding yourself requires that you recognize your own preferences and assumptions about the problem, and that you do not let your emotions cloud your decision-making as you work through the steps. You need to be unbiased, logical, and objective as viewed by your board, your colleagues, your staff, your patients and community, and other stakeholders. You need to step outside of yourself as you view the problem and how it might be solved. This includes always asking yourself if you might be part of the problem.

Understanding your stakeholders requires that you actively seek out and listen to stakeholders affected by the problem to understand their perspectives, perceptions, and feelings of how it is affecting them and how they think it could be resolved. You ask thoughtful, probing, respectful questions in a nonjudgmental way, exhibiting compassion and empathy as you engage with them.

Divergent thinking occurs in two different phases of the Problem-Solving Method to help you avoid jumping to solutions. Divergent thinking during the Define phase ensures that your problem definition thoroughly captures all of the interrelated components of the problem. Divergent thinking during the Study phase requires brainstorming a range of possible root causes and potential alternative solutions to encourage creativity in your final recommended actions that will solve the problem.

PROBLEM-SOLVING METHOD OVERVIEW

As seen in Figure 2.1, the Problem-Solving Method comprises three phases—Define, Study, and Act—each of which has three major steps. A brief overview of the method follows Figure 2.1, and the remainder of the chapter provides an in-depth description of each step and its substeps. Although the Problem-Solving Method shows the steps sequentially, applying the Problem-Solving Method involves cycling back to previous steps as problem-solving progresses.

The letter of each step in Figure 2.1 corresponds to the first letter of that phase, that is, D1 is the first step in the Define phase, S1 is the first step of the Study phase, and A1 is the first step of the Act phase, and so on. Each of the steps has substeps, which are in turn numbered, for example, D1.1 is the first substep of Define step D1.

There are several words that are underlined in Figure 2.1, including Situation, Difficulties, Problem Areas, Issue Statement, Problem Statement, Findings, Conclusions, and Recommendations. These words have very specific meanings in the Problem-Solving Method, as shown in Table 2.1.

DEFINE

D1. Situation & Scope	D2. Stakeholders, Difficulties, & Problem Areas	D3. Issue Statements & Problem Statement
D1.1 Describe the *situation* D1.2 Scope the work	D2.1 Begin stakeholder analysis D2.2 Identify *difficulties* D2.3 Group difficulties into *problem areas*	D3.1 Create *issue statement* for each problem area D3.2 Create overall *problem statement* and vision for future

STUDY

S1. Root Causes & Alternative Solutions	S2. Decision Criteria, Research, & Findings	S3. Conclusions
S1.1 Generate possible root causes S1.2 Generate potential alternative solutions	S2.1 Develop decision criteria S2.2 Determine additional information needed S2.3 Develop *findings* through research S2.4 Review, reflect, and revise approach	S3.1 Collate, analyze, and judge the alternative solutions S3.2 Synthesize judgments into a set of *conclusions*

ACT

A1. Recommendations & Milestones	A2. Communication Strategy & Consensus Building	A3. Implementation & Monitoring
A1.1 Create integrated set of *recommendations* A1.2 Develop key implementation milestones	A2.1 Revisit stakeholder analysis A2.2 Create communication plan A2.3 Implement communication plan and validate approval/consensus of recommendations	A3.1 Develop detailed implementation plan A3.2 Monitor results against key performance indicators

FIGURE 2.1 The Problem-Solving Method.

TABLE 2.1 The Problem-Solving Method Definitions

Situation	The Situation is a description of the difficulties that indicate there is a difference between "what is" and "what ought to be," along with the context of the situation and the key stakeholders involved. The situation can be as short as a passing conversation in the hallway or a written summary of several paragraphs.
Difficulties	Difficulties are the facts, data, and key stakeholders' opinions that identify or imply a gap, or difference, between what the situation is, and what it ought to be. If the difficulty is an opinion, it needs to be stated whose opinion it is, so that facts can be clearly differentiated from opinions. Stick to the facts, data, and stated opinions when listing difficulties. Do not speculate about root causes or alternative solutions in this step.
Problem Area	Each Problem Area is created by grouping interrelated difficulties that identify an important focus for resolution, and assigning a name to that problem area based on the theme of the difficulties it includes. Difficulties can be grouped into more than one problem area. There should be no more than a handful of problem areas.
Issue Statement	Each problem area requires an Issue Statement, written in the form of a key question that needs to be answered to resolve the difficulties in that problem area. The typical format is *"How can (or how should) organization x achieve goal y in light of constraint z?"* The goal in the Issue Statement establishes what ought to be achieved if its set of difficulties is resolved. As such, the Issue Statement is not a yes/no question, a process question, or a question of fact. Rather, it is a key question that leads to exploration of action-oriented alternative solutions that could achieve the goal in the issue statement. A well-written Issue Statement should result in agreement among all stakeholders that this is in fact the key question that needs to be addressed. *The Issue Statement should never have a solution embedded in it.*
Problem Statement	The Problem Statement is a synthesis of all of the issue Statements that summarizes them completely, cogently, and concisely. Its format is also in the form of a question, typically beginning with *"How can"* (or *"How should"*). It also includes the stakeholders that need to be satisfied by the solution, and the major constraints that must be considered in solving the problem. A well-written Problem Statement should result in agreement among all stakeholders that the questions posed in it are the comprehensive set of key issues that need to be resolved to solve the problem. *The Problem Statement should never have a solution embedded in it.*
Findings	Findings are facts, data, and people's opinions or values that are stated as such (along with their underlying rationale for that opinion), that you collect and analyze while doing research. Findings offer the evidence about the root causes of the difficulties and the evidence about the potential alternatives relative to your decision criteria. *The Findings must exclude your personal judgments and values.* You need to ensure that all relevant findings are included, not simply those that support your preferred alternative solution and negate alternatives you do not prefer.
Conclusions	Conclusions are statements that synthesize your judgments about the merits (pros and cons, advantages and disadvantages) of the alternative solutions relative to your decision criteria based on your distillation, synthesis, and interpretation of your research findings. Conclusions justify your preferred alternatives based on your interpretation of your findings, and provide the logic trail of your thought process that links your findings to your recommendations.
Recommendations	Action-oriented Recommendations are your final set of preferred alternatives based on your conclusions across all of the problem areas. Recommendations should be stated succinctly in an action-oriented format. They should be reviewed to ensure that they are consistent across each other, and that as a set, they resolve the difficulties in each of the problem areas identified earlier in the problem-solving process.

■ **DEFINE PHASE SUMMARY**

Define Step D1: The Define phase begins with step D1 with a description of the *situation*. Based on the situation description you develop, you determine the scope of work you will perform given the situation and the time frame available to study and solve the problem. The situation description also identifies the key stakeholders who are affected by the problem.

Define Step D2: You next conduct a stakeholder analysis in Define step D2 by interviewing the key stakeholders to better understand their perceptions and perspectives about the problem. Their opinions, combined with other preliminary facts and data you uncover in these first steps of the Define phase, are the *difficulties*. You list out all of the difficulties and then group them into *problem areas* based on similarity. You then assign a name to each problem area that succinctly describes the theme of its difficulties. You will have at most a handful of problem areas.

Define Step D3: Next, in Define step D3, for each problem area, you write an *issue statement*, which identifies the key question that must be answered to resolve the problem area's difficulties. Finally, you synthesize these issue statements from all of the problem areas into an overall *problem statement*. This is your definition of the problem. Finally, you articulate a vision that describes the organizational goal that will be achieved if the problem is successfully resolved.

■ **STUDY PHASE SUMMARY**

In the Study phase, you work through the Problem-Solving Method problem area by problem area.

Study Step S1: In Study step S1, for each problem area, you brainstorm possible root causes for its difficulties, and identify a range of potential alternative solutions that might resolve the difficulties.

Study Step S2: In Study step S2, you develop the decision criteria by which you will judge the merits of the potential alternative solutions. This delineates the information you need to collect in your research. Conducting your research includes talking to experts, stakeholders, and others in your network of contacts, reviewing relevant literature and websites, and collecting and analyzing additional data. Based on your research, you develop *findings*, or facts, about what you have learned. Once you have completed your research, you review your progress and revise it if necessary.

Study Step S3: You then organize and summarize your findings in Study step S3 to develop your judgments in order to draw *conclusions* about the relative merits of the potential alternative solutions. Your conclusions lead to your recommended course of action to solve the problem in the Act phase.

■ **ACT PHASE SUMMARY**

Act Step A1: In Act step A1, you synthesize your conclusions from across your problem areas into an integrated set of action-oriented *recommendations* that solve the problem. Additionally, you develop an overview of key implementation milestones to facilitate an understanding of overall timeframes and resources needed for implementing the recommendations.

Act Step A2: In Act step A2, you determine the communication and presentation strategy needed to gain approval of the recommendations.

Act Step A3: Once approved, Act step A3 requires that you develop a detailed implementation plan for the recommended actions, and once implemented, their impact must be measured and monitored to ensure they have solved the problem as defined.

The remainder of this chapter describes each of these steps and substeps in detail.

DEFINE PHASE

The Define phase takes you through the first wave of divergent and convergent thinking as you work to understand and define the problem (Figure 2.2). It comprises three major steps, each with several substeps: D1, Situation and Scope; D2, Stakeholders, Difficulties, and Problem Areas; and D3, Issue Statements and Problem Statement. By the time you have completed this phase, you will have defined the problem in the format required by the Problem-Solving Method and articulated a vision for the future that describes the organizational goal that will be achieved if the problem is successfully solved.

DEFINE STEP D1: SITUATION AND SCOPE

Define step D1 describes the situation and determines the scope of work (Figure 2.3). This step summarizes the difficulties that are occurring in the organization that need attention, and how much time and resources will be expended to study and resolve the situation.

DEFINE SUBSTEP D1.1: DESCRIBE THE SITUATION

The <u>situation</u> is a description of the difficulties—facts, empirical data, and key stakeholders' opinions—that indicate there is a difference between "what is" and "what ought to be," along with the context of the situation and the key stakeholders involved.

You cannot correct a situation that hasn't been defined, and you cannot define the real problem to be corrected if you cannot first accurately describe the situation. The purpose of describing the situation is to obtain clarity in the difficulties that need to be corrected.

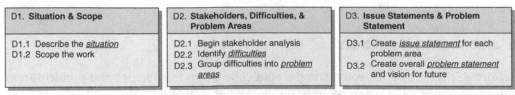

DEFINE

D1. **Situation & Scope**	D2. **Stakeholders, Difficulties, & Problem Areas**	D3. **Issue Statements & Problem Statement**
D1.1 Describe the *situation* D1.2 Scope the work	D2.1 Begin stakeholder analysis D2.2 Identify *difficulties* D2.3 Group difficulties into *problem areas*	D3.1 Create *issue statement* for each problem area D3.2 Create overall *problem statement* and vision for future

FIGURE 2.2 The Define phase of the Problem-Solving Method.

DEFINE

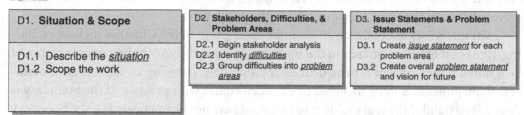

D1. **Situation & Scope**	D2. **Stakeholders, Difficulties, & Problem Areas**	D3. **Issue Statements & Problem Statement**
D1.1 Describe the *situation* D1.2 Scope the work	D2.1 Begin stakeholder analysis D2.2 Identify *difficulties* D2.3 Group difficulties into *problem areas*	D3.1 Create *issue statement* for each problem area D3.2 Create overall *problem statement* and vision for future

FIGURE 2.3 Define step D1: Situation and scope.

You begin the Define phase by briefly describing the situation being faced by the organization as you understand it early on in the problem-solving process. The situation description is the set of facts, data, and opinions derived by conversation, interview, email, memorandum, report, data analysis, or hearsay that relate to the problem being addressed. It may be a combination of various items received from various sources of information, it may be a one-sentence message received over the telephone or a brief hallway conversation, or it may be performance data that are tracked by the organization on an ongoing basis. The situation description also includes a brief background of the context in which these difficulties are occurring, and the key stakeholders involved in the situation.

As you start the problem solving process, the situation description should be succinct. If you are developing a written situation description, it will be no more than about one to three pages in length. As you develop your situation description, it is important to differentiate facts from stakeholders' opinions. Any opinions in the situation should be stated as opinions. As you dig deeper into the problem to understand the context, difficulties, and stakeholders in future steps of the Problem-Solving Method, you may need to cycle back to revise your situation description. By obtaining all pertinent opinions and empirical facts, the need for administrative action is accurately documented in the situation description.

In any given situation, you also need to recognize the context or environment in which the difficulties lie. For example, if the situation involves a healthcare delivery organization that also has an insurance product, how does this context affect the situation? You may not know the answer to these environmental factors as a student or early graduate, but you need to identify them to do some upfront research through reading or talking with your network of professional contacts to gain contextual knowledge. As you gain experience as a leader in healthcare administration, the context will become more intuitive to you as you develop crystallized intelligence with regard to your professional body of knowledge.

As a novice problem solver, you should develop a written situation description to gain expertise in synthesizing the relevant information you are learning about the problem. As you gain experience, you will be able to synthesize the information of the situation description in your head, and you likely will not write it out unless it is a particularly complex situation.

After you have developed a description of the situation, review it to make sure it is complete, and that you really understand it. Does the situation involve a preponderance of short-term or long-term issues? Does this situation involve mostly operational, strategic, financial, policy, or some other type of issues? How much time is available before a decision is needed—an hour, next week, a month from now, three months? What can be accomplished in that time frame in solving the problem?

Common errors in obtaining an accurate description of the situation include excluding important opinions or facts of the situation, or conversely, including ones that should be ignored if the problem is to be defined appropriately. Drawing an appropriate boundary of the difficulties to be included or excluded comes with practice. If the boundary is drawn "too tightly" the real problem to be solved may not be uncovered. If the boundary is "too loose," the focus of the problem solving process may be lost.

DEFINE SUBSTEP D1.2: SCOPE OF WORK

The scope of work is the portion of the overall situation that needs to be addressed now. The scope must be clear in terms of breadth, depth, time frame and expected end product. Depending on the situation, you may also need to include a clear articulation of budget and any organizational resource constraints that affect the completion of the scope of work.

Defining the scope of work will entail some initial data collection to help determine what can or should be included or excluded in the scope given the time frame and the breadth and depth of the expected end product. In many cases, it will be impossible to immediately address all of the difficulties in a given situation in a particular time frame. At other times, a portion of the problem might be excluded in the scope for a number of valid reasons. This substep allows you to pause and make a conscious decision to include or eliminate parts of the situation for consideration at this time.

View the scope of work from two perspectives, both breadth, and depth. That is, what areas should be studied or not studied, and how deeply should each area be explored? In addition, consider time allocation and the number of team members involved. You need to balance the amount of resources and time you can devote to this particular situation in light of other current needs, responsibilities, and demands of your time and attention, your team or staff, and your organization. The expected end product also makes it clear whether the expectation now is to identify the problem only, propose multiple alternatives, choose the best alternative, implement the choice, or resolve it. The time frame for these gradations of scope makes a real difference.

As you move forward in solving the problem, you may find something new that has implications for what might need to be added or deleted from the scope. In this case, the scope can be adjusted, either expanded or contracted.

In summary, in scoping the work, you need to be sure you are clear on:

- The scope of the difficulties to be corrected (depth and breadth, and what to include or exclude)
- Your understanding of the objectives of your problem solving efforts and the product to be delivered (e.g., report, presentation)
- The due date for the deliverable
- The amount of time to be allocated (and if relevant, budget, resources required, etc.)

DEFINE STEP D2: STAKEHOLDERS, DIFFICULTIES, AND PROBLEM AREAS

In Define step D2 you (a) begin the stakeholder analysis, (b) identify the difficulties, and (c) group the difficulties into problem areas (Figure 2.4). This is a key step of the Define phase, as it is where you must fully embrace the "never assume" principles and engage in divergent thinking to "make the problem bigger." This includes always asking yourself during this step if you are part of the problem.

DEFINE SUBSTEP D2.1: BEGIN STAKEHOLDER ANALYSIS

Based on the situation description, you begin to identify and list persons internal and external to the organization who are involved in and/or affected by the problem in some way. These people are called stakeholders. And, the person or persons to whom your deliverable will be provided and approved, and any persons who will be responsible for implementing the recommendations or affected by them, are also stakeholders. In healthcare delivery, patients, their families, and the community should always be considered stakeholders, because whatever problem is being experienced in the organization will impact them in some way. As you progress into later steps of the Problem-Solving Method, other stakeholders will come to light. When that happens, you will circle back to this substep to add them to the stakeholder list.

The information you collect from the stakeholders during your interviews includes their perceptions, perspectives, and feelings about the situation, including:

- Their view of the situation
- How it is affecting their work environment
- How they operate in the situation or process (observe the process if possible)
- What they see as key difficulties
- What they view as possible root causes for these difficulties
- What their suggested alternative solutions are and why
- What their goals are for getting the problem as they see it resolved

In addition, some of the stakeholders will be able to provide you with organizational documents, data, reports, financial statements, or other secondary data that will be useful

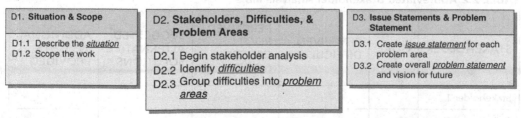

FIGURE 2.4 Define step D2: Stakeholders, difficulties, and problem areas.

to you in future steps of the Problem-Solving Method. Or, they may provide you with recommendations for other people or groups internal and external to the organization who could provide you with useful insights and information as you work through the steps of the Problem-Solving Method.

After completing each interview, you review your interview notes and summarize your results into a table format that facilitates your ability to analyze what you have discovered through your interviews. This is called a *stakeholder analysis*. The stakeholder analysis also helps you understand how the stakeholders will need to be engaged with over the course of the project, which is covered in the communication strategy of the Act phase of the Problem-Solving Method (Step A2). An abbreviated example stakeholder analysis table is shown in Table 2.2. The number of rows would be expanded to the number of stakeholders in the situation.

As described in Chapter 1, a "never assume" attitude requires that you engage in divergent thinking when conducting a stakeholder analysis. You must listen to each stakeholder with an open mind. You do not argue with them or tell them they are wrong, even if you think their view is incorrect. You do need to ask probing questions to their replies to make sure you understand their underlying rationale or reasoning for what they are telling you. Stakeholders often frame problems in terms of preferred solutions (e.g., we need more staff). When this occurs you need to ask follow-up questions to ensure you understand why the stakeholder holds this view. What is their goal that their preferred solution would help them achieve? What is it that not having enough staff is preventing them from doing? These conversations with stakeholders help you step outside of yourself to be able to view the problem from all different points of view.

Your stakeholder analysis helps you:

- Identify the various stakeholders relevant to the situation
- Describe the difficulties in the situation that they perceive as needing correction
- Gain initial information on the relative priority of the difficulties needing correction, the time frame in which they must be corrected, and the resources available to correct them
- Identify the goals, objectives, and standards which aren't being achieved or maintained as perceived by the various stakeholders, and verified by data where possible, and whether the goals, objectives, or standards are derived from social, organizational, personal, management, employee, or other sources

TABLE 2.2 Abbreviated Stakeholder Analysis Table

STAKEHOLDER	GOAL	PERCEIVED DIFFICULTIES	PERCEIVED ROOT CAUSES (WHY?)	SUGGESTED ALTERNATIVE SOLUTIONS	ADDITIONAL INSIGHTS PROVIDED
Stakeholder 1					
Stakeholder 2					

- Determine whether there is an absence of agreement on the appropriate goals, objectives, and standards among the stakeholders, disagreement as to whether the goals, objectives, and standards are being achieved, and disagreement as to the prioritization of the goals and objectives

- Gain insights into existing or potential interpersonal conflict among the stakeholders, including whether you are part of the problem

- Identify secondary data sources, including reports, financial statements, and other quantitative data to gain empirical evidence about the situation

- Identify possible root causes of why the difficulties are occurring, both as perceived by the stakeholders and verified by available data

- Identify preliminary solutions to the problem as perceived by the stakeholders and others, including what should be done by whom, when, where, how, and why

- Identify who will be the final decision-maker regarding what is an acceptable solution

- Determine who will need to be involved in implementing the final solution and who will be affected by it

Common errors in conducting a stakeholder analysis include:

- Assuming that the opinions gathered are facts. Be sure to separate facts from opinions by cross checking against other stakeholders' opinions and empirical data. A stakeholder's opinion that is assumed to be a statement of fact can lead to solving the wrong problem.

- Lumping stakeholders with different views of the problem into the same stakeholder group. For example, in a given situation, the Emergency Department physicians may have a very different view of the problem than the Admitting physicians. Their responses should therefore be on different rows in the stakeholder analysis table.

- Accepting suggested alternative solutions identified by stakeholders and other key informants as the only potential alternatives considered later in the Problem-Solving Method. Listen to what the stakeholders say regarding their preferred alternative solutions, but you must expand beyond those alternatives when you get to the Study phase of the Problem-Solving Method.

- Not recognizing that you may be part of the problem. Unless you have clear evidence to the contrary, you should always examine whether your actions and behaviors or lack thereof are causing difficulties.

DEFINE SUBSTEP D2.2: IDENTIFY DIFFICULTIES

Difficulties are the facts, data, and key stakeholders' opinions that identify or imply a gap, or difference, between what the situation is and what it ought to be. In order for an opinion to be a fact, it has to be stated in the difficulty whose opinion it is.

Based on data, facts, and opinions you have collected so far, you engage in divergent thinking by identifying and listing the difficulties. You collect as many difficulties as time allows by conducting the stakeholder analysis, reviewing organizational data, and if possible, direct observation of the situation.

All difficulties must be true, factual statements. You will have empirical data and other facts that are indisputably true at this point in time. But, at this step, you do not know whether the opinions that have been provided by stakeholders are true or accurate. And you will very likely have differing opinions among your stakeholders.

If difficulties must be true, how then can you state these opinions as difficulties? Someone's opinion can be stated as a fact by writing in the difficulty whose opinion it is. Even if you do not personally agree with a stakeholder's opinion, you must include it as a difficulty. You do not insert your judgment into this phase, but as part of divergent thinking, keep an open mind and create a numbered list of all the difficulties presented to you by stakeholders or discovered through data analysis or observation.

Do not speculate about root causes or potential solutions when defining the difficulties—just state the facts of the problem. At this substep, you assemble a list of as many difficulties as possible in the time available to you, and you do not pass judgment on any of them. This is a substep in the Problem-Solving Method that is helping you "make the problem bigger" by preventing you from prematurely narrowing in on just a subset of difficulties.

When talking with stakeholders, it can sometimes be confusing to differentiate their stated difficulties from their root causes and preferred solutions. For example, an operating room nurse may tell you that the reason operating room flow is poor is because the scheduler is incompetent, and the scheduler should be fired. This nurse has revealed to you a belief about a possible root cause of the problem—the scheduler is incompetent, and a solution to that hypothesized root cause—fire the scheduler. But, the nurse has also revealed an opinion that should be stated as a fact to make it a difficulty—the operating room nurse believes the scheduler is incompetent.

At this substep in the Problem-Solving Method, you do not know for a fact that the scheduler is incompetent. So, writing the difficulty as "*the scheduler is incompetent*" is not correct. But it is a known fact at this point in time that "*the operating room nurse stated that the scheduler is incompetent*." This is a difficulty, because it is a fact that the operating nurse stated this as their opinion. Remember, all difficulties must be facts. At this substep in the Problem-Solving Method, it does not matter whether the stakeholders' perceptions are accurate. It is in the Study phase that you will investigate whether the perceptions are accurate.

To better define what is to be corrected or improved, the problem solver should determine:

- What organizational purposes, goals, objectives, standards, values, or customer needs and expectations are not being met? Is there agreement among the stakeholders?
- What are the precise difficulties needing correction or improvement? Are they validated by opinion and empirical evidence?
- Which are the more significant difficulties?

Common errors in identifying difficulties include:

■ Forgetting that for an opinion to be stated as a fact, it needs to be stated in the difficulty whose opinion it is.

■ You personally speculating in this substep about root causes, preferred alternatives, or anything else that comes later in the Problem-Solving Method.

■ Not recognizing that you or your behavior may be a difficulty and/or a root cause. Are you letting your experience or judgment cloud what you include or exclude as difficulties? Are you lacking self-awareness of whether you are causing difficulties? You always need to ask yourself if your behaviors or actions may be contributing to the problem.

DEFINE SUBSTEP D2.3: GROUP DIFFICULTIES INTO PROBLEM AREAS

A problem area is a grouping or "bucket" of interrelated difficulties that identify an important focus for resolution. Each problem area is given a name or label that captures the theme of its difficulties.

In this substep, you begin to engage in convergent thinking by developing a classification scheme for your difficulties. To do this, you separate them into different "buckets" based on how similar they are to each other. These "buckets" are the problem areas. The goal is to converge on no more than a handful of problem areas for a situation. Generally, you will end up with between three and five problem areas, although the number of problem areas to be used is based on personal judgment.

Grouping difficulties into problem areas is not a hard and fast science, but comes with experience. There are different strategies for grouping difficulties. You can organize difficulties based on a common subject, for example, financial versus strategic issues. Or you can group difficulties based on an objective or set of objectives identified by stakeholders that relate in common to that set of difficulties. Or a logical grouping of difficulties may relate to a possible common root cause, which if eliminated, would rid the organization of that set of difficulties.

Although a difficulty can be placed in more than one problem area, the goal is to try to have the problem areas as independent of each other as possible. This makes the problem-solving process manageable by breaking the problem into mutually exclusive problem areas that can be solved semi-independently of the other problem areas.

This doesn't mean the problem areas are completely independent. Rather, it is analogous to identifying the subsystems (i.e., the problem areas) in a larger system (i.e., the problem) such that the links within each subsystem are much stronger than the links between them.

You then look at the set of difficulties in each problem area, and attach a name or label to it based on the theme the difficulties in that problem area seem to represent. Labels could be "clinic workflow," "provider relations," or "leadership accountability," for example. You should *not* first create a list of problem area names and then force difficulties to fit within it. This could result in a Type III Error—solving the wrong problem. The name for each problem area should flow from its difficulties. The problem areas should be specific enough to ensure that all difficulties are being addressed, but broad enough to provide a smooth uncluttered flow of the problem-solving thought process.

There are no right or wrong ways to group the difficulties. So how do you know if your problem areas are in the most helpful buckets possible before moving to the next step of the Problem-Solving Method?

One way is to review all of your problem areas and your stakeholder analysis. Is there a possible root cause identified in the stakeholder analysis that tends to underlie multiple problem areas? If so, it may signal that the problem area groupings need to be rethought, such that the difficulties that may have the same underlying possible root cause are grouped into the same problem area. This is because if your subsequent research identifies that these difficulties did have the same actual root cause, eliminating that root cause would likely eliminate most, if not all, of those difficulties.

If your problem areas contain a lot of overlap, you may find in the Study phase of the Problem-Solving Method that the same list of potential alternative solutions may be relevant to multiple problem areas. If this happens, you would likely benefit from circling back to your problem areas to see if they could be revised to be more mutually exclusive of each other.

Common errors in grouping difficulties into problem areas include:

- Creating too many or too few problem areas. Group similar difficulties such that you end up with no more than a handful of problem areas as a rule of thumb.

- Grouping difficulties such that there is a great deal of overlap between the problem areas. If you find in the Study phase that the same possible root causes or potential alternative solutions keep appearing across multiple problem areas, your problem areas may have too much overlap between them. You should revisit your problem areas to see if you can make them more mutually exclusive of each other.

DEFINE STEP D3: ISSUE STATEMENTS AND PROBLEM STATEMENT

In Define step D3, you engage in convergent thinking to identify the key issue in each problem area that needs to be addressed if the problem is to be resolved. Then, to define the problem, you synthesize the issue statements into an overall problem statement that also indicates the key stakeholders that must be satisfied by the solution to the problem (see Figure 2.5).

Issue statements and problem statements are written in the format of action-oriented questions, that if answered, would make the difficulties in the problem area dissipate or disappear. It takes practice and higher-order thinking skills to state the key issues completely and concisely

DEFINE

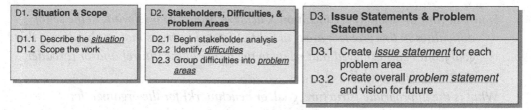

FIGURE 2.5 Define step D3: Issue statements and problem statement.

Successful problem-solving requires asking the right questions. If you are working with a team in solving a problem, a lot of your time, focus, and discussion should be on this step. The purpose is to develop written issue statements and a written problem statement that all stakeholders agree are the key questions that need to be answered to solve the problem.

DEFINE SUBSTEP D3.1 CREATE AN ISSUE STATEMENT FOR EACH PROBLEM AREA

An issue statement is the key question that needs to be answered to eliminate, correct, or resolve the set of difficulties in its problem area. An issue statement is required for each problem area. It leads to exploration of action-oriented alternative solutions to resolve that problem area's set of difficulties.

When you get to Define step D3, you have at most a handful of named problem areas, each with its set of related difficulties. In this first substep, you pause and consider the rationale behind why you grouped the difficulties into these respective problem areas. What is the goal for each problem area? What are the constraints that are preventing that goal from being achieved?

Asking yourself these questions helps you articulate the key issue that needs to be addressed in each problem area if its difficulties are to be resolved. The purpose of articulating the issue for each problem area is to provide guidance as to what must be studied in the Study phase of the Problem-Solving Method to find the best acceptable solution to resolve each problem area's difficulties.

An issue statement is written in the form of a question, usually starting with the words "*how can*" or "*how should*," although it sometimes also starts with the word "*what*." As you develop the question, you consider what the goal for the problem area is that should be achieved if the difficulties identified in the problem area were eliminated. Additionally, you determine what are the barriers or constraints that are keeping that goal from being achieved and/or the broader organizational goals that should be considered when choosing a course of action.

The format of an issue statement helps identify the key question that needs to be addressed in each problem area. They are written in a way that invites exploration of a range of potential action-oriented alternative solutions that could resolve the problem area's difficulties in order to achieve the goal of the problem area.

Some typical formats of an issue statement are:

How can (or how should) organization X achieve {stated goal relevant to the set of difficulties in this problem area} in light of {stated barriers that are hindering that goal from being achieved that relate to the vision of the future} and/or {broader organizational goals}?

What is the appropriate {structure, goal, or benchmark} for the organization regarding {problem area focus}, and how can the organization best achieve that {structure, goal, or benchmark} in light of {stated barriers} and/or {broader organizational goals}?

Each issue statement establishes the goal that ought to be achieved if the set of difficulties in its problem area is resolved. The issue statement is structured such that it mandates an action-oriented mode of thinking. A well-stated issue needs to clearly and succinctly identify the key question in the problem area. However, it should be specific enough to the situation at hand that anyone reading the set of issue statements would have a clear sense of what is going on without reading the situation description you developed in Define substep D1.1.

An issue statement is *not* a rhetorical or esoteric question, a yes/no question, a process question, a research question or a question about facts.

And *an issue statement should never contain a solution*. If an issue statement is framed as a solution, it prematurely closes off divergent thinking about other alternative solutions that could eliminate the set of difficulties in the problem area when you get to the Study phase. For example, if an issue is framed as "How can we hire more nurses to improve quality of care?" you have closed off from consideration a plethora of other potential alternative solutions that might improve quality of care. The only solution under consideration with this wording is the one embedded in this issue statement—hire more nurses.

Once all the issues have been identified (one issue statement per problem area), a decision must be made as to whether there is a logical ordering to the issues, and whether some issues are long term versus short term in their time horizon. The "central issue" is derived by ordering the priority of issues across the problem areas. The central issue is the "first" in this list; the one that is key to resolving the others. Another way to determine the "central issue" is: If the other issues are resolved but the "central issue" is not, then the problem is no nearer a solution than *not* resolving the other issues. This naturally leads to a priority listing of the issues.

When working with a team to solve problems, the debate should be focused on writing the issue statements. Writing issue statements invites discussion among the team members to arrive at the key question to be answered for each problem area. This helps focus the discussion on what is the right question, which keeps the discussion from immediately and prematurely jumping to an unproductive argument at this phase of problem-solving as to what is the right solution. A well-written issue statement should result in agreement among all team members and key stakeholders that each issue statement is, in fact, the key question that needs to be addressed in its problem area.

It takes practice to write an issue statement that accurately identifies the key question that needs to be addressed. Mastering this substep demonstrates your ability to not just collect facts—the difficulties—but to be able to synthesize and integrate the facts to understand, develop, and articulate the key issues that need to be addressed in the problem areas. You have taken what is "the mess" of the problem, and have broken it down into its component parts—the problem areas. And, you have identified the key issue in each problem area.

The important points to remember regarding issue statements are: (a) the issue should be stated in the form of the key question that needs to be answered to resolve the difficulties; (b) the question leads to exploring action-oriented alternative solutions; and (c) the issue statement should never contain an alternative solution embedded in the question.

By the conclusion of this substep, you should have developed an issue statement for each problem area, identified which issues are short and long term, the order of importance of the issues to the organization, and the priority for study. The priority for study may be different from the order of importance of the issues depending on the time available, or the immediate needs of the organization, for example.

The most common errors in writing issue statements are:

- Not framing the issue as a key question, but instead writing a question as a yes/no question, or asking about facts that can be discovered through research.
- Embedding a solution in the issue statement.
- Neglecting to study and review your set of issue statements to determine the priority order of the issues, particularly if one of the issues seems to be the "central" issue, the answers to which will impact the answer to the issue statements of the other problem areas.

DEFINE SUBSTEP D3.2: CREATE AN OVERALL PROBLEM STATEMENT AND VISION FOR THE FUTURE

The <u>problem statement</u> is a complete, concise, and cogent summary, synthesis, and integration of the issue statements that also enumerates the key stakeholders that need to be satisfied by the solution, and the major constraints that must be considered in solving the problem.

The final substep of the Define phase completes the first wave of convergent thinking in the Problem-Solving Method by writing the problem statement.

Writing the problem statement is the culmination of the preceding substeps, particularly the issue statements. The problem statement summarizes, synthesizes, and integrates the issue statements across your problem areas completely, cogently, and concisely, yet is thorough enough to cover all aspects of the problem. In addition, it includes the stakeholders that need to be satisfied by the solution, and the major constraints that must be considered in solving the problem.

The problem statement statement is also written in the form of a question that typically begins with "*how can*" or "*how should*" or "*what.*" And, just like the issue statements, the problem statement is not a yes/no question, a process question, or a question of facts, and it should never have a solution embedded in it. Example formats for the problem statement follow:

> *How can (or how should) organization X achieve {stated goals synthesized from across the issue statements} in light of {stated barriers in the issue statements} and/or {broader organizational goals} to the satisfaction of {list of key stakeholders in the situation}?*

> *What is the appropriate {structures, goals, or benchmarks as identified in the issue statements} for the organization regarding {key issues}, and how can the organization best achieve the {structures, goals, or benchmarks} in light of {stated barriers summarized from across the problem areas} and/or {broader organizational goals} to the satisfaction of {list of key stakeholders in the situation}?*

Here you begin to appreciate the skill and importance of writing the problem statement. A problem stated too simply does not weigh all factors needing consideration. However, a problem statement that is too long and has too much detail will just be confusing, not illuminating. Initially, you may feel like you are engaging in an exercise of developing the art of the run-on sentence when trying to synthesize the issue statements into an overall problem statement, but that is okay. With time, you become more expert in writing clear, cogent, and succinct problem statements.

The purpose of a problem statement is to enable the problem solver to step back from the individual issues and consider them in their interrelationship to each other. This synthesis is crucial because it may identify that the critical issue may be found *between* problem areas.

For example, one problem area may deal with an issue of how to best achieve better access to care, while two other problem areas may deal with issues of how to improve provider relations and leadership accountability. In combination, the most critical issue facing the organization may be how to best resolve the problem areas simultaneously, while keeping in mind the organizational goals and vision for the future. For example, the problem statement might be:

> *How can we improve access to services while simultaneously enhancing provider relations and leadership accountability, in light of the organization's commitment to the quadruple aim and vision to be the community's preferred place to receive healthcare services, and to the satisfaction of our patients, their families, the community we serve, and our employed and network providers?*

The problem statement should capture these interrelationships and how they relate to the vision for the future, and the stakeholders that are most affected by the problem.

When working with a team, writing the problem statement invites discussion among the team to come to agreement that these key questions in the problem statement are the ones that must be answered to successfully solve the problem, and that no key stakeholders have been forgotten. The problem statement should help the team answer the question: "What is really the problem here—what are the critical issues we are trying to resolve in this situation?"

Then the team should ask themselves: "If we solve this problem as framed in this problem statement, will we correct the situation? Are we on the right track given our vision for the future?" Skillful leaders excel at facilitating their teams through the Define phase of the Problem-Solving Method to help them arrive at a well thought out, mutually agreeable problem statement. If the team works through the Define phase of the Problem-Solving Method successfully, the probability of committing a Type III error—solving the wrong problem—is minimized.

The last part of this substep is to clearly articulate the vision for the future in the context of the problem statement. If all of the key issues in the problem statement were successfully resolved, what would be the impact on the organization? This helps answer the "why" question to all stakeholders of what you are trying to achieve by solving this problem. In addition, the vision for the future provides a beacon toward which your organization is moving as it solves the multitude of problems that arise. Without this beacon, problem-solving can devolve into reactive decision-making. You do not want today's solution to a problem to become tomorrow's problem. Writing the vision for the future helps you keep thinking ahead, and places your problem-solving efforts within the broader strategic context of the organization.

STUDY PHASE

Once you have an agreed upon a problem statement, you are ready to begin the Study phase of the Problem-Solving Method. The Study phase takes you through a second wave of divergent and convergent thinking as you study each problem area (Figure 2.6). It comprises three major steps: S1, Root Causes and Alternative Solutions; S2, Decision Criteria, Information Needs, Research, Findings, and Review; and S3, Conclusions. Each of these steps has several substeps.

Generally, you work through the Study phase steps on each problem area individually. The exception is that when you complete Study substep S2.3, Develop findings through research, you will look across all of your information needs to develop an integrated research plan to collect your findings across your problem areas. This is because you may need to ask a content expert or stakeholder a set of questions during your research that spans multiple problem areas. You want to be able to talk with that expert once to ask all of your questions across your problem areas. You do not call them to ask your questions for one problem area, then call them again to ask your questions related to another problem area, and so on.

STUDY

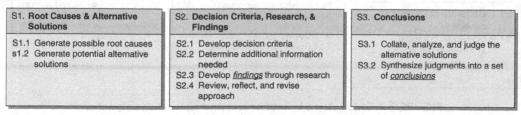

S1. Root Causes & Alternative Solutions	S2. Decision Criteria, Research, & Findings	S3. Conclusions
S1.1 Generate possible root causes s1.2 Generate potential alternative solutions	S2.1 Develop decision criteria S2.2 Determine additional information needed S2.3 Develop *findings* through research S2.4 Review, reflect, and revise approach	S3.1 Collate, analyze, and judge the alternative solutions S3.2 Synthesize judgments into a set of *conclusions*

FIGURE 2.6 The Study phase of the Problem-Solving Method.

As you gather your findings through research, you will circle back to record your notes in the appropriate places of your tools or tables described in the substeps that follow specific for each problem area. This helps you organize your notes and understand what you have learned and what information may still be missing.

By the end of the Study phase, you will have generated and researched possible root causes and alternative solutions for each problem area, and then judged the relative merits of the alternatives against your decision criteria to arrive at conclusions about which alternatives are preferred based on the findings from your research.

STUDY STEP S1: ROOT CAUSES AND ALTERNATIVE SOLUTIONS

Up to this point in the Problem-Solving Method, you have focused on facts. In this first step of the Study phase, you now are allowed to extend beyond facts to hypothesize about what might be causing the difficulties in the problem areas, and what alternative solutions might modify, alleviate or eliminate the root causes (Figure 2.7).

STUDY SUBSTEP S1.1: GENERATE POSSIBLE ROOT CAUSES

Understanding the possible root causes of the difficulties leads to the development of alternative solutions to eliminate, avoid, or modify them, thus correcting or improving the difficulties they are causing.

You began identifying possible root causes in Define substep D2.1 during your stakeholder analysis. For example, during your stakeholder interviews, the operating nurse told you their opinion that the scheduler is incompetent (a possible root cause) and should be fired (a potential alternative solution). Thus, you begin this Study substep already having some ideas about possible root causes from your work in prior steps of the Problem-Solving Method. These are your starting set of possible root causes.

In this substep, you build on your initial set of possible root causes as part of divergent thinking to identify additional possible root causes. The goal is to generate as large a set of possible root causes as feasible to facilitate brainstorming a variety of potential

STUDY

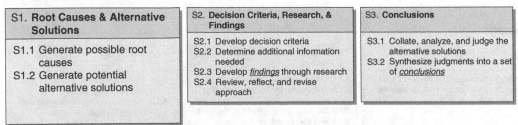

FIGURE 2.7 Study step S1: Root causes and alternative solutions.

alternative solutions to address those possible root causes that are explored during your research in the Study phase step S2.

An initial approach in identifying additional possible root causes is to look at your difficulties, as they are "symptoms" of the underlying problem. But, just as resolving symptoms in medicine doesn't cure an underlying disease, addressing only the symptoms that are the difficulties will not eliminate the problem. You need to brainstorm about the possible root causes of the difficulties.

For each difficulty, you should ask yourself why that difficulty might exist. You then ask why your answer exists, repeating several times to get to what is called the "5th order why" in root cause analysis. As you probe more deeply by asking "why," you get closer to identifying the underlying possible root cause.

In addition to generating possible root causes by looking at your difficulties, there are other ways to generate them. These include observing the part of the organization experiencing the problem, analyzing organizational data relevant to the problem area, and reading the literature for publications that discuss other organizations that have experienced a similar problem.

You need to keep an open mind about possible root causes as you conduct your research into the problem in the Study phase step S2. As you engage in research, you will uncover additional possible root causes, which means you need to circle back to this step and add them to your list. At this step of the Problem-Solving Method, you do not know which are the actual root causes. Thus, your possible root causes represent hypotheses to be explored in Study substep 2.3, where you develop findings through your research.

Common errors in generating possible root causes include:

- Neglecting to identify, question, and analyze root causes at all. This error will lead you to solve the wrong problem by addressing symptoms without fixing the real cause of the difficulty.

- Assuming that the first possible root cause you identify for a difficulty is the only possible root cause to investigate. You must dig farther down into successive levels of asking why a difficulty exists to get to the underlying possible root cause.

- Not continuing to be on the alert for additional possible root causes as you move forward into the research step of the Study phase.

- Not recognizing that your behavior or actions may be a possible root cause of a difficulty.

STUDY SUBSTEP S1.2: GENERATE POTENTIAL ALTERNATIVE SOLUTIONS

Divergent thinking continues when you generate potential alternative solutions that would eliminate, avoid, or modify the possible root causes you identified in the previous substep. Alternative solutions are different possible answers to the "how" part of the question posed in the issue statement. As such, they should be action-oriented, not process oriented. Thus, "collect more data" is not an alternative solution. Potential alternative solutions need not be mutually exclusive.

And, "do nothing" is an action—an alternative to take no action—that maintains the status quo for the time being. Sometimes after studying the issue in detail, you might conclude that nothing should be or can be done to resolve that issue at this time, with justifiable reasons for maintaining the status quo. Thus, an alternative solution is always to do nothing—maintain the status quo. But, of course, you cannot decide at this point in the problem-solving process if "do nothing" would be the best acceptable alternative. But it should always be included as an alternative solution to be considered through research.

The process of generating potential alternative solutions began when you collected ideas about suggested alternative solutions from the stakeholders when you conducted your stakeholder analysis in the Define phase substep D2.1. You should include all of these potential alternatives in your list to be studied. This is because when you get to the Act phase of your recommendations, you must be able to provide the logic for the justification of why a preferred alternative by any given stakeholder did not make it to the final set of recommended actions.

In this substep, you are now expanding the list of potential alternative solutions beyond what you learned during your stakeholder analysis. Remember that you are still engaging in divergent thinking when generating potential alternative solutions. As part of divergent thinking, you do not judge any of your generated potential alternative solutions at this time. At this substep, you do not think in terms of "right" or "wrong" solutions, but in terms of "alternative" solutions. There are no pre-existing right or wrong alternatives. You brainstorm as many as possible.

Another important point when generating potential alternative solutions is that in your mind, you may think that it is highly unlikely that one of your alternatives could be successfully implemented. Remember, keep engaged in divergent thinking. The alternative should stay on the list as a potential alternative so that it is researched, but you should also think about the alternatives that could be implemented in the short-term that could move you toward that more comprehensive alternative.

When generating additional potential alternative solutions, you need to have the courage, imagination, and creativity to arrive at novel alternatives. Do not assume at the outset that the wildest solution cannot be done, and do not worry at this substep as to what is the "best" versus the "best acceptable" solution. The difference between "best" and "best acceptable" is that when you get to the research step of the Problem-Solving Method, you may find that the "best" solution cannot be implemented, so you will have to default to the "best acceptable" solution if you want an alternative that can be successfully implemented. The important thing to remember is to be imaginative, developing possibilities specific for this problem and not using some checklist of prior known or taught solutions.

There are a number of ways to generate ideas for additional potential alternative solutions, including looking at your root causes for ideas about what alternatives could eliminate them, searching the literature and the Internet to identify benchmark alternatives, talking with your network of colleagues or experts in the field, thinking about alternatives for both the short term and the long term, and engaging in creativity exercises to identify innovative alternatives. Once you have developed your list of potential alternative solutions across your problem areas, you should review them as a total set to ensure that the list is comprehensive, creative, and action-oriented. If you discover more potential alternatives when you get to the research substep S2.3 of the Study phase, you should circle back and add them to your list.

STUDY STEP S2: DECISION CRITERIA, RESEARCH, AND FINDINGS

In step S2 of the Study phase, you first develop decision criteria that will be used to judge the merits of the potential alternative solutions you generated. This will drive the information you need to collect to determine how the alternative solutions compare on these criteria.

Based on the information you need, you develop the questions you need to research to develop facts, called findings, about the possible root causes and the potential alternatives. You develop a consolidated research plan from your information needed across your problem areas, and then conduct your research.

When you have completed your research, you take a deliberate pause to review and reflect upon your work so far, and determine if you need to circle back to earlier steps of the process for revisions (Figure 2.8).

STUDY SUBSTEP S2.1: DEVELOP DECISION CRITERIA

By this step of the Problem-Solving Method you have a list of possible root causes with their accompanying list of potential alternative solutions. In Study substep S2.1 you develop decision criteria against which you will judge your potential alternative solutions. Your decision criteria support the Study phase in a couple of ways. First, they help you identify what you will need to know to choose among your potential alternative solutions, which helps you articulate the information you will need to gather (Study substep S2.2).

Second, the decision criteria help you articulate what will be required for successful outcomes and implementation of the potential alternative solutions within the context of this

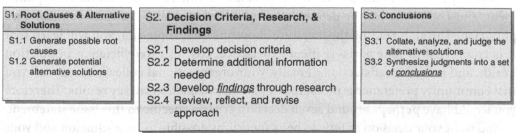

STUDY

S1. Root Causes & Alternative Solutions	S2. Decision Criteria, Research, & Findings	S3. Conclusions
S1.1 Generate possible root causes S1.2 Generate potential alternative solutions	S2.1 Develop decision criteria S2.2 Determine additional information needed S2.3 Develop *findings* through research S2.4 Review, reflect, and revise approach	S3.1 Collate, analyze, and judge the alternative solutions S3.2 Synthesize judgments into a set of *conclusions*

FIGURE 2.8 Study step S2: Decision criteria, research and findings.

situation and your organization. Remember that your goal in the Study phase is to draw conclusions about the best acceptable alternatives, not the best alternative. If the best alternative solution cannot be implemented successfully, then you will not have resolved the difficulties and solved the problem. Hence, you need to strive for the best acceptable alternatives.

Skipping criteria development could become a fatal mistake in the problem-solving process. A shortcut might lead you to recommend a solution that has no chance of being successfully implemented. The criteria posed must be comprehensive to ensure you will solve the problem effectively, but they must also be limited only to those that are needed to solve the defined problem.

What criteria should you consider to judge your alternative solutions? Typical decision criteria that are relevant for many problem areas' alternative solutions include fit with the organization's culture and mission, vision, and values; fit with broader community needs or context; legal compliance and ethical considerations; timeframe required to implement; cost to implement and maintain; innovativeness; and stakeholder preferences. For example, if you are dealing with a crisis situation, it is important that an alternative can be implemented quickly to stem the crisis. Thus, the timeframe required to implement the solution would be a relevant decision criteria in this situation.

In addition to these typical decision criteria, you should review the issue statement to identify other decision criteria specific to the goals and constraints or context in it. The constraints or context are generally found in the part of the issue statement that comes after the "in light of" portion of it. For instance, suppose the issue statement is as follows:

How can we improve access to and continuity of outpatient services in light of the organization's commitment to the quadruple aim and its vision to be the community's preferred place to receive healthcare services?

Given this issue statement, there are three broad phrases that stand out: access to and continuity of outpatient services, quadruple aim, and community preference. In this instance, you would need criteria that can be used to define access to and continuity of outpatient services. You would also need criteria that define the quadruple aim, as well as community preference.

If you do not have experience in this situation, you may not know what relevant criteria might be used for these three broad phrases. Thus, as a novice, you may need to read relevant literature and talk to colleagues and experts in this area to get a better understanding of what criteria should be considered.

You may find, for example, that access is usually defined as wait time for an appointment, and continuity can be defined as patients being able to see their primary care physician. Through reading the literature about the quadruple aim, you will learn that it is comprised of four parts—patient experience, cost of care/efficiency, population health, and provider satisfaction.[1] Finally, your organizational colleagues may tell you that community preference is measured by patient satisfaction survey results. Therefore you would have perhaps around seven decision criteria specific to this issue statement.

You want your decision criteria to be as specific as possible to your situation and your organization. This is because what might be the best acceptable alternative solution in another organization may be completely disastrous in yours. The same problem could exist in two different organizations, but different contexts within them, such as organizational mission, vision, values, culture, financial pressures, heavy managed care penetration, or physician leadership, might require a completely different solution in each organization. For example, solutions requiring heavy financial investment may not be preferred in an organization that is near bankruptcy. In such a case, financial feasibility would be an example of a decision criterion that would be relevant when assessing the merits of any alternative solutions for that organization.

Once you have identified your decision criteria, you should create a decision criteria table to organize your decision criteria and your potential alternative solutions in a matrix format. In the table, the left hand cell of each row lists an alternative solution, while the top cell of each column lists a decision criteria. You create a decision criteria table for each problem area. An abbreviated version of a problem area decision criteria table is shown below in Table 2.3.

At this substep, all of the other cells in the decision criteria table are blank, because you do not have the information you need yet to describe the alternatives relative to the criteria. Once you have completed your research in Study substep S2.3, you will be able to summarize your findings in the appropriate cells of the table. As you conduct your research in the Study substep S2.3, you may need to come back to this table to add new alternative solutions or additional decision criteria.

Things to remember as you develop decision criteria include:

- Make sure you understand the territory—what is the history, culture, climate, and environment of this organization? Pay attention to the things that have been historically important to the organization; for example, political, cultural, financial, public, ethical, legal, demographic or marketplace considerations, and any special needs of stakeholders. These organizational contexts can have implications for the decision criteria that should be used to judge alternatives.

- Determine what "type" of case you are facing to aid you in identifying decision criteria—is this primarily a case about mergers, process flow, human resource issues, union issues, reorganization? If so, you should read literature and talk to experts about the implications for decision criteria.

- Look back at the stakeholder analysis to determine if there are any needs in that problem area not being met. If there are, this may indicate adding a decision criterion to capture this unmet need.

TABLE 2.3 Problem Area Decision Criteria Table

PROBLEM AREA A	CRITERION 1	CRITERION 2	CRITERION 3	CRITERION 4
Alt Solution 1				
Alt Solution 2				
Alt Solution 3				

STUDY SUBSTEP S2.2: DETERMINE ADDITIONAL INFORMATION NEEDED

You need to conduct research about each of the potential alternatives relative to each of the decision criteria. Before you carry out your research, you need to identify what additional information you need to guide your research efforts. The additional information needed are the questions you will need to have answered through your research.

The focus of Study substep S2.2 is to generate as questions the additional information you need, for which you will get answers through your research in Study substep S2.3. Then, in the Study phase step S3, you will summarize, collate, and review the information you have collected during your research to develop your judgments and draw conclusions about actual root causes and which alternative solutions are preferred. Your conclusions will then inform your recommended course of action in the Act phase of the Problem-Solving Method.

The questions you develop as you identify the additional information you need are questions of facts, data, and experts' opinions and rationale for those opinions. For example, for an issue statement with a goal of ensuring access to care, suppose one of your potential alternative solutions is to increase urgent care availability. The information you need to know for this alternative relative to the decision criteria might be:

- How much additional urgent care capacity would need to be added? Is that cost-effective relative to other options to increase outpatient capacity?
- If more urgent capacity is added, where should it be located in our market?
- How would additional urgent care capacity impact continuity of and access to outpatient care?
- Would urgent care improve the quality of outpatient care, and if so, how?
- How do primary care physicians feel about their patients going to urgent care as opposed to seeing them? Are there other alternatives to urgent care that primary care physicians prefer more?
- How do patients and the community feel about urgent care access compared to seeing their primary care physician or other outpatient options?
- What are patient satisfaction scores for and comments about our current urgent care offerings?

As you determine the questions to identify the information you need in each problem area, you will need to determine what additional internal and external data you will need to analyze, whether you need to observe any work processes, whether you need a better understanding of the context of the problem, whether you need additional information from any stakeholders, and whether you understand the history and culture of the organization relative to the problem.

You may also see that a key issue in the problem area may be a particular problem "topic," for example a merger issue. You would want to read literature about that key issue topic to learn if there are topic-specific questions you should be asking as part of your research to ensure you get the information you need.

Once you have developed all of your research questions across your problem areas, you organize them into one integrated research plan. List out all of your questions into one document, and then organize them based on the source you will use to get them answered. This will facilitate and streamline your research process.

Your research questions can be answered by more than one source. Sources to get your questions answered include interviews, reading the literature and relevant reputable websites, and analyzing data and reports. Persons to interview include stakeholders and content experts and colleagues both internal and external to the organization. Literature to review can include articles in both academic and trade journals. Websites can include those of relevant professional organizations and consulting companies. Data needs might be facts about the external environment, as well as relevant data internal to the organization.

STUDY SUBSTEP S2.3: DEVELOP FINDINGS THROUGH RESEARCH

Findings are the facts discovered through your research that offer evidence for or against possible root causes and the acceptability of potential alternative solutions based on your decision criteria.

Although information is gathered in all phases of the problem-solving process, it is during this substep that the data collection process is most comprehensive. You use the research plan you developed in the previous substep as the guide to conduct your research in this substep.

In this substep of the Problem-Solving Method, you focus on discovering indisputable facts through your research that, when synthesized, constitute your findings. The purpose of collecting these facts is to identify actual root causes of the difficulties, and to help you make judgments and draw conclusions to rule in or rule out alternative solutions in the Study phase step S3 of the Problem-Solving Method.

Findings are statements of fact, people's opinions or values that are stated as such (along with their underlying rationale for that opinion), and data that you collect and analyze while doing research. In addition to conducting interviews and reading literature and websites, the application of data analytics, statistical models, financial analyses, market analyses, and the like are often necessary during this substep of the Study phase.

Findings offer the evidence in each problem area for or against the possible root causes and the alternative solutions relative to the decision criteria. *Although findings can include others' values and opinions as long as it states whose they are, they cannot include your values and opinions.* You must set your values and opinions aside while you conduct your fact finding.

As you conduct your research, you will often uncover new difficulties or problem areas, additional stakeholders, and new ideas around possible root causes and potential alternative solutions. If you do, you should cycle back and update and revise your work in the previous steps of the Problem-Solving Method. If you uncover something that indicates the potential for a major change in the scope of work, you will need to talk with the person to whom you are reporting to discuss whether the scope should be changed.

When doing research to discover your findings, you need to match the time available to the appropriate level of data gathering and analysis. Paralysis by analysis should be avoided. Recognize that you will never have perfect information to make a decision, but you must have enough relevant data to convincingly inform your ultimate conclusions and recommendations about the best alternatives to pursue.

As you develop findings through your research, you will discover that some possible root causes will prove to be unfounded based on the evidence. When this happens, any alternative solution that was generated to address only that root cause is also not supported. Thus, some evidence you collect will both eliminate a possible root cause, and its associated alternative solution.

For example, you may find through your research that the operating room scheduler is well respected for their expertise by the majority of stakeholders you interviewed. This would lead you to conclude in substep S3.2 that the possible root cause of scheduler incompetence is not supported. This finding would, in turn, eliminate its associated potential alternative solution of firing the scheduler.

In the course of conducting your research, you will discover many findings that end up having little relevance to your alternative solutions under consideration. You do not include these irrelevant facts in your research summary. Instead, the findings you include should be limited to those that are significant to reaching conclusions on the best acceptable solution(s) to the problem. Thus, the findings record the facts particularly important to guiding the decision as to the appropriate solution to the problem.

On the other hand, you cannot exclude from your findings those that are relevant to choosing among alternative solutions, but that you do not personally like. You must include all relevant findings, even if they provide evidence for an alternative solution you do not personally like, or provide evidence against your preferred alternative. In other words, you cannot "cherry pick" your findings to fit your preferred alternatives. Infusing the findings you present with your personal bias is unethical and could result in reaching faulty conclusions in support of a solution being implemented that ends up being disastrous for the organization.

STUDY SUBSTEP S2.4: REVIEW, REFLECT, AND REVISE THE APPROACH

By the time you reach this substep of the Problem-Solving Method, you have defined the problem, generated possible root causes and potential alternative solutions, and conducted research to develop findings. As you have worked through the Problem-Solving Method's steps and substeps, you will likely have had to circle back to previous ones for revision as you learned more the further you progressed into the Problem-Solving Method.

Study substep S2.4—Review, reflect, and revise the approach—is inserted as a "hard stop" to encourage you to go back and look at all of your work so far. This is the point where you will especially want to review your problem areas. Based on all of your work so far, particularly in what you are learning through your research, do these "buckets" still make sense? Are they comprehensive or did you discover a new set of difficulties along the way that would rise to adding another problem area? If so, is the work represented by the new set of difficulties and problem area significant enough that it requires going back to renegotiate the scope of work?

Additionally, review your issue statements. Are the key questions posed in the issue statements still relevant and do they seem logical to the alternatives that have been explored? Do you feel confident that the findings you have collected can now answer those questions, or are there still holes in what you need to know? And are there still holes in your alternatives and decision criteria that suggest a more diversified range of alternatives need to be explored to answer the key questions in your issue statements?

Another key step in reviewing your work is to go back to your stakeholder analysis. Given what you have found through your research, are some alternatives rising to the top tier for becoming preferred solutions? Are those the solutions that are preferred by your stakeholders? By some stakeholders and not others? What might you need to communicate back to your preceptor, boss, or key stakeholders at this point in the process? You should set up meetings with key stakeholders at this step to gain feedback, validation, and logic checks on your work so far.

This communication achieves at least two goals. First, it ensures you are circling back to check your logic before you get too far down the line. Second, it keeps your key stakeholders informed of what you are thinking. By the time you get to your recommendations, there should be no surprises among the key stakeholders about what your recommendations will be. And, for you, there should be no surprises as to what the reactions will be by key stakeholders to your recommendations. Keeping them informed at major touch points along the way helps avoid unwanted surprises and resistance to your final set of recommendations later in the Problem-Solving Method.

STUDY STEP S3: CONCLUSIONS

By the start of Study phase step S3, you will have a comprehensive set of notes from your research. These notes are facts about possible root causes and the potential alternative solutions relative to the decision criteria. These notes may include other people's opinions about the best course of action and why, identified by whose opinions they are to make it a research fact. But they should not include *your* opinions, preferences, or judgments because you need to keep the facts separate from your judgment. Everyone looking at your research findings should be able to agree that these are the facts.

But different people looking at the same set of facts may arrive at different conclusions. It is in this step, Study step S3, that you develop *your* judgments and conclusions (Figure 2.9). You need to organize your notes into a format that supports your ability to review them to make judgments and draw conclusions about what you have learned. Thus, this is the step where you apply your logic.

To facilitate your ability to do this, you organize your notes into the appropriate cells of the decision criteria table. The cells that are at the intersection of each alternative and each decision criteria should contain your relevant research facts.

STUDY

S1. **Root Causes & Alternative Solutions**	S2. **Decision Criteria, Research, & Findings**	S3. **Conclusions**
S1.1 Generate possible root causes S1.2 Generate potential alternative solutions	S2.1 Develop decision criteria S2.2 Determine additional information needed S2.3 Develop *findings* through research S2.4 Review, reflect, and revise approach	S3.1 Collate, analyze, and judge the alternative solutions S3.2 Synthesize judgments into a set of *conclusions*

FIGURE 2.9 Study step S3: Conclusions.

You then review those facts to apply *your judgments* to what you have learned. Your judgments are your assessments about the pros and cons and strengths and weaknesses of the alternatives relative to the decision criteria. Finally, you synthesize your judgments into an overall set of conclusions about which alternative solutions are preferred and why.

STUDY SUBSTEP S3.1: COLLATE, ANALYZE, AND JUDGE THE ALTERNATIVE SOLUTIONS

You now have in front of you copious notes you have taken through your research to arrive at your findings. In this substep, you will organize and analyze your findings about the alternatives relative to the decision criteria to help you systematically judge the merits of the alternative solutions.

First, review all your findings and organize (collate) them into each relevant alternative-decision criteria cell of the problem area decision criteria table (see Table 2.4). You complete a separate table for each problem area. Up to this point, everything in the table is factual. The table assembles your findings as indisputable facts on which there should be common agreement among your team and key stakeholders. Your logic, opinions and values should not be in any of the table's findings.

Rarely will any one alternative rise to the top above all others across all of the decision criteria. Some alternatives will be better on some criteria, but worse on others. So, your findings will almost never reveal a clear-cut "winning" alternative. Instead, deciding on the best course of action based on the findings will entail having to make trade-offs.

This is where your judgment now comes into play. You will review and analyze your table of findings to arrive at *your judgments* about the relative merits (pros and cons and strengths and weaknesses) of each alternative relative to the decision criteria. Your

TABLE 2.4 Problem Area Decision Criteria Table With Findings

PROBLEM AREA	CRITERION 1	CRITERION 2	CRITERION 3	CRITERION 4
Alt Solution 1	Relevant Findings	Relevant Findings	Relevant Findings	Relevant Findings
Alt Solution 2	Relevant Findings	Relevant Findings	Relevant Findings	Relevant Findings
Alt Solution 3	Relevant Findings	Relevant Findings	Relevant Findings	Relevant Findings

judgments are based on applying your logic, values and opinions to the evidence in the table. Depending on the situation, you may want to develop a scoring method that weights the decision criteria and assigns points to the findings to develop a numeric value for each alternative to facilitate your thought process about the trade-offs you are making in judging them.

Because judgments are based on personal logic, values, and opinions, two different people can look at the same set of evidence and arrive at different judgments about the merits of the alternatives. This means there may not be common agreement in interpreting the findings. That is why it is important to first collate findings—indisputable facts on which there is agreement—before you make judgments about the relative merits of the alternatives, for which there may not be agreement. It is often helpful to summarize your judgments as a new column in your completed decision criteria table (Table 2.5).

STUDY SUBSTEP S3.2: SYNTHESIZE JUDGMENTS INTO A SET OF CONCLUSIONS

Conclusions are statements that synthesize your judgments about the relative merits of the potential alternatives, and which are preferred or not, based on your distillation, synthesis, and interpretation of the findings.

In this substep, you engage in convergent thinking to "hone in" on which alternatives are your final preferred set. Based on the findings and your judgments about the relative merits of the alternatives, you will synthesize your judgments into a set of conclusions for each problem area that rule in and rule out the potential alternative solutions. This ruling in and ruling out of alternatives by problem area, and your rationales, are your conclusions. Two people may look at the same set of facts, yet arrive at different judgments and conclusions about the preferred course of action.

Which alternatives rise to the top, and why? Which are less desirable, and why? Your findings are statements of fact. Your judgments are your views about the pros and cons of the alternatives based on your findings. Your conclusions are your holistic statements

TABLE 2.5 Problem Area Decision Criteria Table With Findings and Your Judgments

PROBLEM AREA	CRITERION 1	CRITERION 2	CRITERION 3	CRITERION 4	YOUR JUDGMENTS
Alt Solution 1	Relevant Findings	Relevant Findings	Relevant Findings	Relevant Findings	Pros/Cons, Strengths/ Weaknesses
Alt Solution 2	Relevant Findings	Relevant Findings	Relevant Findings	Relevant Findings	Pros/Cons, Strengths/ Weaknesses
Alt Solution 3	Relevant Findings	Relevant Findings	Relevant Findings	Relevant Findings	Pros/Cons, Strengths/ Weaknesses

about the set of alternatives that were explored and a synthesis of what alternatives are preferred versus not preferred, and why, based on your judgments.

Conclusions are not simply restating all of your judgments. Rather, they are a synthesis of your judgments into, at most, a handful of statements for each problem area that summarize your logic and justification for alternatives being rules in or ruled out.

Conclusions stop short of recommendations, which comes in the Act phase of the Problem-Solving Method. Conclusions should be thought about as the logic trail that links your findings and judgments to your recommendations. As a rule of thumb, anyone reading your conclusions should have a pretty good idea of which alternative solutions will end up as your recommended ones.

Recall that the problem statement in the Define phase includes the phrase that the problem must be solved "to the satisfaction of {list of key stakeholders}." This does not mean that each stakeholder group will get their preferred alternative solution. What it means is that the stakeholders know their preferred alternative was researched, they accept as fact the evidence you collected about that alternative, and they accept as sound your judgments and conclusions for why their preferred alternative is not in the organization's best interest to pursue. This is especially important for stakeholders who may have veto power or who will be responsible for implementing your recommendations.

As you review your conclusions about the relative merits of the alternative solutions, go back to review your stakeholder analysis about the various stakeholders' preferred alternatives. Is there a key stakeholder whose preferred solution is not going to rise to the set of recommended ones? Is there an alternative solution to which a key stakeholder was opposed, but your conclusion is that it is preferred? If so, your evidence (findings) and judgments and conclusions will need to be convincing. Are your findings solid? Are your judgments and conclusions sound?

ACT PHASE

The Act phase of the Problem-Solving Method entails creating action-oriented recommendations that flow logically from your conclusions, and developing a strategy that supports their successful implementation.

Once accepted, the recommendations require a detailed implementation plan and associated metrics to close the loop of the problem-solving process by ensuring the recommendations as implemented have solved the problem (Figure 2.10).

ACT

A1. **Recommendations & Milestones**	A2. **Communication Strategy & Consensus Building**	A3. **Implementation & Monitoring**
A1.1 Create integrated set of _recommendations_ A1.2 Develop key implementation milestones	A2.1 Revisit stakeholder analysis A2.2 Create communication plan A2.3 Implement communication plan and validate approval/consensus of recommendations	A3.1 Develop detailed implementation plan A3.2 Monitor results against key performance indicators

FIGURE 2.10 The Act phase of the Problem-Solving Method.

ACT STEP A1: RECOMMENDATIONS AND MILESTONES

In Act step A1 of the Problem-Solving Method, you recommend the action-oriented alternatives that flow from your conclusions, and describe key milestones that are required to implement them. At this step, you integrate your recommendations across all of your problem areas so that you are presenting one integrated set (Figure 2.11).

ACT SUBSTEP A1.1: CREATE AN INTEGRATED SET OF RECOMMENDATIONS

Recommendations are an integrated set of action-oriented solutions that answer the questions posed in the issue statements and problem statement while simultaneously moving the organization toward its vision for the future.

Each problem area has its own set of conclusions. You now synthesize the conclusions about your preferred alternative solutions across all of the problem areas into one set of action-oriented recommendations.

The action-oriented recommendations are the final set of preferred alternative solutions that flow from your conclusions across all of the problem areas. They are the answers to the questions posed in the issue statements and the problem statement. Because recommendations are action-oriented, they should start with a verb. Recommendations should be stated succinctly, and it should be clear what action is being requested.

Recommendations should be reviewed to ensure that they are consistent across each other, and that as an integrated set, they resolve the root causes of the difficulties in each of the problem areas. You must be able to show that the recommendations solve the problem as defined, and close the gap between "what is" and "what ought to be."

Your logic trail linking your findings, conclusions, and recommendations must be clear. The recommendations should be prioritized in order of importance, and the sequence and timing of the recommendations should be clear and justified. The recommendations must be well understood by all stakeholders, and you must be able to demonstrate and defend that they solve the problem as defined.

It is important to circle back to the issue statements and the problem statement, paying particular attention to the constraints articulated in them, such as budget or

ACT

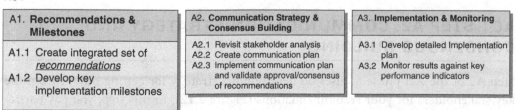

A1. Recommendations & Milestones	A2. Communication Strategy & Consensus Building	A3. Implementation & Monitoring
A1.1 Create integrated set of *recommendations* A1.2 Develop key implementation milestones	A2.1 Revisit stakeholder analysis A2.2 Create communication plan A2.3 Implement communication plan and validate approval/consensus of recommendations	A3.1 Develop detailed Implementation plan A3.2 Monitor results against key performance indicators

FIGURE 2.11 Act step A1: Recommendations and milestones.

time frame. You need to double check that your recommended solutions are feasible given these constraints. If they are not feasible, then they will not solve the problem as stated.

This gets back to the notion that the "best" alternative may not be possible. You need to ensure that your alternatives are the "best acceptable" in closing the gap between "what is" and "what ought to be" to the satisfaction of key stakeholders given the constraints in the issue statements and problem statement. Your goal is to arrive at the best acceptable solutions that can actually get implemented given the stakeholders, the time frame, the budget, the organizational culture, and other constraints in the situation.

Note that "to the satisfaction of key stakeholders" does not mean that all stakeholders get what they want, or that only recommendations preferred by stakeholders should be put forward. Because the goal of problem-solving is implementing recommendations that fix the problem, stakeholders must come to agreement that the proposed recommendations are, in fact, the best acceptable course of action for the organization at this point in time.

As part of your stakeholder analysis and research process, you have learned what stakeholders' preferences are, and what opposition they may have to certain recommendations. If a recommendation that is opposed by certain stakeholders is in the best interest of the organization, your role as a leader is to put forth that recommendation with a clear, logical justification of why it is the best alternative, along with a strategy and implementation plan that convinces stakeholders that it is the best course of action, regardless of their personal preferences.

ACT SUBSTEP A1.2: DEVELOP KEY IMPLEMENTATION MILESTONES

Decision makers who will approve your recommendations must understand at a high level the financial and resource obligations implementation will place on the organization. And those who will be involved in implementing the solution must fully understand their role and the major steps they must take to fulfill their obligations.

To ensure the successful implementation of your solution, it is essential that the overall high level plan for implementing the solution and the resources required are clear. This high level plan should include key implementation milestones, which are the major steps, and their related resource requirements and timelines that will be required to implement your recommendations. They are *not* a detailed implementation plan, which comes in the final step of the Act phase.

ACT STEP A2: COMMUNICATION STRATEGY AND CONSENSUS BUILDING

Step A2 of the Act phase focuses on developing a strategy for getting buy-in from the key stakeholders for your recommendations (Figure 2.12). In this step, you pay particular attention to laying out your presentation strategy and formulating any final written

ACT

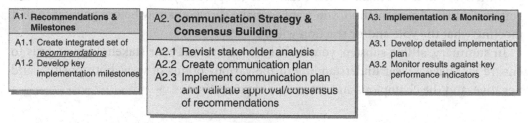

FIGURE 2.12 Act step A2: Communication strategy and consensus building.

report, and strategically communicating with your stakeholders throughout the problem-solving process.

This requires a well-thought out communication plan that you develop based on your understanding of your key stakeholders. The goal is to get your stakeholders to approve either formally, when a vote is required, or through consensus, when a vote is not required, to move forward with the recommendations.

ACT SUBSTEP A2.1: REVISIT STAKEHOLDER ANALYSIS

Reviewing your stakeholder analysis is the first step in developing a communication strategy. You need to refresh your memory of the different viewpoints of the stakeholders, and think about how those viewpoints will likely influence their reactions to your recommendations. Which ones will likely favor them? Oppose them? Who might be the champions? The detractors? Thinking about these questions will help inform the communication plan you should develop to build consensus and mitigate any resistance to the set of recommendations developed.

A key goal of this substep is for you to anticipate scenarios of how certain individuals or groups may respond to your recommendations based on the stakeholder analysis. Based on this, you build specific touch points into the communication plan to anticipate this response and address them along the way, before the recommendations go before any formal body for approval. Not all recommendations will go through a formal approval process, but knowing and addressing stakeholder viewpoints is important in this scenario, as you will need to build consensus to move forward with success and to sustain the recommendations and execution of the implementation plan.

Remember that you also revisited the stakeholder analysis in the Study phase to determine the key stakeholders with whom you should meet to review your problem-solving work. Thus, communicating with key stakeholders at regular intervals happens throughout the problem-solving process, and not just at this current substep.

You should have been receiving feedback along the way. This does not mean that you discard any recommendations that one or more stakeholders oppose. It means that you get their feedback and continue to explore how the recommendations might be re-shaped or re-communicated to gain the necessary approval.

If there are decision makers who must vote to approve your recommendations after you give a formal presentation, you want to make sure you know before going into that meeting what the vote and/or reaction will be.

In summary, at this substep, you circle back and revisit your stakeholder analysis to ensure you have a clear understanding of the various points of view, both positive and negative, and the champions and detractors of your efforts.

ACT SUBSTEP A2.2: CREATE A COMMUNICATION PLAN

Different stakeholder groups require different levels and types of information provided to them in different formats. Therefore, your communication goals with each of these groups will likely be different.

In order to reach a collective understanding, consensus, or a "yes" vote, it will be important for you to develop a communication plan to keep stakeholders informed. Although this substep appears toward the end of the Problem-Solving Method, the sophisticated problem solver will start to formulate this communication plan earlier rather than later in the process.

A communication plan identifies the key stakeholder groups with whom you need to communicate, the message, format, and time frame for communicating with those stakeholder groups, and your overall objectives of communicating with them.

The communication plan you develop provides you with an overall summary that describes the steps needed to gain approval or consensus of the plan to date. Any communications that are needed to support the later step of implementing recommendations would be included in the implementation plan versus in your communication plan. The focus of this substep is to anticipate the goal of the communication along with the "who, what, when, and where" that is needed to move the recommendations forward in terms of acceptance and approval.

The stakeholders who are key for successful implementation will need regular updates. You never want the key decision-making stakeholders to be surprised by your final set of recommendations. Keeping them regularly informed along the way helps avoid a situation in which your recommendations are not accepted.

By this substep in the process, you want to pay particular attention to how you formulate any formal written deliverable, and your presentation strategy to gain approval or consensus of your recommendations. Other stakeholders may need less intensive or personal communication, such as regular email communication instead of meetings.

Implementing the communication plan usually involves a presentation to various approval bodies or teams that need to vote or build consensus to move forward. Presentation skills, meeting management, a strong public relations/communication team partner and emotional intelligence are key during this substep.

Of particular importance is your presentation strategy to the key stakeholders who have either formal voting authority or informal decision-making power regarding moving forward with the recommendations. Your recommendations should invite action. The action should invite understanding, commitment, and a "yes" vote to the proposed solution by the stakeholders who have the right to decide. The key stakeholders should have been brought along throughout the entire problem-solving process. Again, there should be no surprises on their end or on your end about what you will be presenting or how the votes will go following your presentation.

As you prepare for your final presentation, you should be clear about the following as you develop your presentation strategy:

- What is the purpose of the meeting—what do you hope to accomplish? The opening remarks of any presentation should grab the audience's attention and also include the end goal of the meeting whether it is consensus on an issue or a formal vote to implement the recommendations.

- Carefully plan the *strategy* of the presentation. It need not be in the same order as your written report, and in fact, it probably should not be. Think about the best way to sell the recommendations to the decision makers present at the gathering. The logical organization of the presentation is key to engaging the listeners and influencing them to say "yes." As part of your strategy, give credit to all who contributed to your efforts. If an alternative that ends up being recommended arose from someone else's idea, say so.

- Know the audience. Does it include the Board, the CEO, physicians, members of the community or the media, your boss? What are they prepared to act on at this meeting? Make sure the key people who support your recommendations will be there. What information will be critical to this audience when considering the recommendations? What details are appropriate for the audience? Cost, convenience for patients and their families, relation to the mission, community benefit, or loss of autonomy might be important factors for different stakeholders.

Sometimes, in spite of your best efforts, it becomes clear during the discussion period of your presentation that your recommendations as currently stated will not get approved. You should anticipate this potential before going into the meeting so that you have thought about a backup compromise contingency plan. You will need to be willing to compromise.

In this circumstance, you need to listen closely to the stakeholders to see if you can get approval of at least a subset of the recommendations so that action can move forward in the organization. What recommendations can be agreed upon now, with further work in the future to gain approval of the remainder of the recommendations?

Finally, the communication plan might include a press conference or statement, written communications sent via email or mail, and web/social media content. The channel and content of the plan would have been developed in the previous substep, and this is the substep in which the plan is executed.

ACT STEP A3: IMPLEMENTATION AND MONITORING

By Step A3 of the Act phase, your recommendations have been approved either by consensus or formal vote, and need to be implemented and monitored to ensure they are having their intended impact in solving the problem as defined (Figure 2.13).

ACT

A1. Recommendations & Milestones	A2. Communication Strategy & Consensus Building	A3. Implementation & Monitoring
A1.1 Create integrated set of *recommendations* A1.2 Develop key implementation milestones	A2.1 Revisit stakeholder analysis A2.2 Create communication plan A2.3 Implement communication plan and validate approval/consensus of recommendations	A3.1 Develop detailed implementation plan A3.2 Monitor results against key performance indicators

FIGURE 2.13 Act step A3: Implementation and monitoring.

ACT SUBSTEP A3.1: DEVELOP A DETAILED IMPLEMENTATION PLAN

Once your action-oriented recommendations have been accepted, they must be implemented. The final test of whether you have successfully solved the problem is if your recommendations actually get implemented and have their intended impact.

For some situations, a detailed implementation plan might simply be each member of the senior leadership team knowing what their action items are when they leave a meeting. But for many organizational problems, implementation usually requires change management skills and, depending on the problem, a highly detailed project management implementation plan, such as a detailed Gantt chart.

Depending on the complexity of the recommendations, successful organizational change management required to implement the recommendations may require involvement from the organization's project management department. The implementation plan must explicitly describe the resources that will be necessary to execute the recommended solutions.

Elements such as the time frame, deliverables, deadlines, personnel required, and financial resources required must all be clearly spelled out. The "owner" responsible for leading the implementation process must also be identified. The details of project management are beyond the scope of this text. For those with an interest in learning more about project management, we refer you to the website of the Project Management Institute (see www.pmi.org).

ACT SUBSTEP A3.2: MONITOR RESULTS AGAINST KEY PERFORMANCE INDICATORS

The problem-solving process does not end with the implementation of the recommendations. You need to know if your recommendations are having their intended impact. What is the organization expecting to see if the problem has been successfully solved with your recommendations?

This should be clear from the stated vision for the future developed in Define step D3. This vision for the future then needs to be translated into a meaningful measure that can be tracked. For example, will patient satisfaction scores improve, and by how much? Will appointment wait times decrease? Will operating margins improve?

Your recommendations will need a set of key performance indicators that define the metrics that should be tracked to measure success, along with how the metrics should be measured and captured for ongoing analysis. Depending on the problem and its magnitude in the organization, some performance indicators may only need to be tracked in the short term until you are certain the improvements have taken hold. In other cases, the key performance indicators may become a part of the organization's formal departmental, service line, or organizational level dashboard of key performance indicators.

Be clear about the time frame needed to see improvement in the performance indicators, and that there is agreement about the time frame. Some indicators may change quickly in response to an action (called lead indicators), while others may need time to see an impact (called lag indicators). What is the needed time frame to see the intended impact?

If the key performance metrics and touching base with key stakeholders indicate the problem has been solved as defined, it still might require periodic evaluation. Many organizational issues tend to recycle themselves. The Problem-Solving Method is a thought process that not only applies to a crisis situation, but as part of a monitoring process to consciously assess organizational performance to identify opportunities for improvement. These inquiry and feedback loops are a critical component of a systematic approach to organizational problem-solving.

EVERYDAY USE OF THE PROBLEM-SOLVING METHOD

At this point, you may be asking, "That's a lot of steps. Do leaders really use this method?" The almost universal answer from the University of Minnesota alumni is:

> Yes, I use the Problem-Solving Method every day. Unless it is a very complex problem, I do not write out the steps as the process is ingrained in me. But I automatically take myself out of the situation to be objective and start to explore the problem.

If practitioners do not use every single step with every single problem they are facing every day, how does the Problem-Solving Method become a natural part of leading and problem-solving?

First is internalizing the principles of "never assume." These principles require that you remain calm, impartial, and logical, stepping outside of the situation as if you were an impartial consultant to avoid your biases influencing your decisions. This is about valuing and listening to stakeholder input, asking the right questions of the right people to understand the problem and ways they think it should be resolved. Finally, it is important that you avoid rushing to solutions, instead taking a broad view of what might possibly be the root causes, and generating a range of potential alternative solutions to alleviate the problem.

Second is internalizing the steps of the problem definition phase of identifying difficulties and grouping them into problem areas as part of your autonomic thought process—just like your nervous system, it just happens in response to stimuli.

You first "make the problem bigger" to avoid developing too simplistic a definition of the problem. In identifying difficulties, you differentiate what is fact, and what is opinion. Accepting opinions as facts is avoided.

Based on the difficulties, you classify the difficulties into meaningful groupings to ensure you have captured all of the "buckets" that are "the mess" of the problem. As you practice this, it is a thought process that can occur automatically in a matter of minutes.

As you gain experience in using the Problem-Solving Method when you begin your healthcare administration career, these steps will become part of your automatic thought process as you carry out your work every day. A colleague, clinician, staff member, boss, or patient or their family member may engage you in a conversation or email about something that indicates there is a difficulty. You will follow up to get further clarification and information to better understand the situation.

Based on that conversation, you will determine who else (other stakeholders) you need to speak with, and what data are readily available for you to look at to better understand the situation. Based on what you hear and see, you will be able to list the difficulties in your head, and in your thought process group them into at most a handful of problem areas.

You will then be able to formulate in your head the key issue that needs to be resolved in each problem area. Depending on the scope of the problem, the issues may be something you can resolve yourself within a short period of time, or you may decide that these issues will require more extensive follow up by a broader team of people. This whole process might take at most 5 to 10 minutes of your time.

So, although these steps may seem time consuming when you first practice them, they become part of your automatic thought process as you master them.

Third, you gain confidence the more you practice the Problem-Solving Method. You are looked at by your peers as wise, because you have developed the ability to quickly identify and look at each problem area, and ask the key question that needs to be answered—the issue statement.

And, in team situations, you model this approach to problem definition to engage the team in productive discussions to come to agreement on what the problem is. This enables all to come to a common, explicitly stated definition of the problem that asks the key questions that need to be answered to solve the problem. The Problem-Solving Method becomes the "reasoning" processor that the organization uses to define and solve problems.

But in using the Problem-Solving Method in everyday problem-solving, you avoid using the "lingo" of the problem-solving definitions, but focus on the Problem-Solving Method's logic.

Fourth, the Problem-Solving Method requires that you recognize the difference between research findings—which are facts on which all must agree; conclusions—which are the synthesis of judgments about the findings; and recommendations—which are action-oriented solutions that resolve the problem, and flow logically from the conclusions.

The Problem-Solving Method helps you develop the ability to listen to other's logic, and tease out whether what you are hearing are facts or their judgments about the facts. Facts are facts. Opinions, judgments, and conclusions are not facts.

Finally, through your stakeholder analysis and communication strategy, the Problem-Solving Method helps you systematically focus on what it will take to get your recommendations implemented and what is the best way to build consensus. Your goal is to "get to yes," and this doesn't happen by accident.

In learning the Problem-Solving Method, you need to master the Problem-Solving Method in its entirety, which requires writing out each step in detail. Parts II, III, and IV of this book will serve as a practice guide to lead you through each of the steps and substeps. As you do so, remember to circle back to this chapter to read the detailed description of the step.

In summary, as you progress in your career, you will begin to automatically use the Problem-Solving Method as your mental "reasoning processor." Just like the example of learning to ride a bike, the steps become coordinated, seamless, and internalized. You will not have to consciously think about the steps. They just come naturally. You will have achieved the master level of becoming a "never assume" problem solver.

REFERENCE

1. Bodenheimer T, Sinsky C. From triple to quadruple aim: Care of the patient requires care of the provider. *Ann Fam Med*. 2014;12(6):573–576. https://dx.doi.org/ 10.1370%2Fafm.1713"10.1370/afm.1713

CHAPTER 3

COMPARISON OF PROBLEM-SOLVING METHODS

We fail more often because we solve the wrong problem than because we get the wrong solution to the right problem.[1]

Russell Ackoff

INTRODUCTION

When you begin working in a healthcare organization, you may learn that they "practice Lean," or they follow principles of "Design Thinking," or they mention some other model of how they approach and solve problems as an organization. This chapter describes how the Problem-Solving Method compares to these two methods. Regardless of the organizational problem-solving method used in the organization, your knowledge of using the Problem-Solving Method as your thought process will be complementary to, and not competing with, these other methods. As described in this chapter, the two aspects of the Problem-Solving Method that will be most useful to you regardless of the problem-solving method used in the organization are how to define the problem and engaging with stakeholders.

This chapter may be more meaningful to you after you have actually practiced applying the steps of the Problem-Solving Method. Thus, you may want to skip to Parts II, III, and IV of the text, and come back to this chapter after you have gained more familiarity in using the Problem-Solving Method.

STRENGTHS OF THE PROBLEM-SOLVING METHOD

There are several problem-solving methodologies widely used in healthcare today. Examples include Lean, the Institute for Healthcare Improvement approach to Quality Improvement (IHI-QI), and Design Thinking. In addition, if you conduct a web search on the term "problem-solving method" or "problem-solving process," an endless number of results are returned—"seven steps for effective problem-solving," "the four basic steps of the problem-solving process," and any number of steps for problem-solving. Regardless of the method proposed, all have the following generic steps in common: define the problem, study the problem, and act on the problem.

The two primary strengths of the Problem-Solving Method presented in this text lie in: (a) how to define the problem, and (b) engaging with and considering stakeholders. As discussed in Chapter 1, "The Problem Is Not Always What It Seems," organizational problems are rarely unidimensional. They comprise several interrelated issues that all need to be resolved to successfully solve the problem. In defining the problem, you need to identify all of these interrelated issues. Otherwise you risk solving the wrong problem.

The approach to defining the problem in the Problem-Solving Method is elegant in its comprehensiveness and simplicity. It does not require extensive training in statistics or any complicated methodologies. It does take practice and discipline to learn so that it becomes the way you automatically think when solving problems. The core elements of defining the problem are:

1. Actively listen to a multitude of stakeholders with an open mind to document their view of the situation and review available relevant data. As you listen to the stakeholders, you listen for the difficulties—the data, facts, and opinions that indicate there is a difference, or gap, between what the situation is, and what it ought to be. Do not make any assumptions about root causes or alternative solutions in this step. If you are working with a written case for a class or a case competition, you identify the difficulties by highlighting them as you read through the case. Look for the sentences or phrases that indicate there is a gap between what is and what ought to be. Be clear in sorting out facts from opinions. Opinions need to state whose opinion it is to make it a fact and to ensure you collect all opinions. Make a list of the difficulties.

2. Go through the difficulties one by one and group them into buckets based on similarity. Although a difficulty can be placed in more than one bucket, try to keep the buckets of difficulties as mutually exclusive from each other as possible. Review the difficulties in each of the buckets and assign a name to the bucket based on the theme of its difficulties. This is a problem area. You should end up with no more than a handful of problem areas.

3. For each problem area, develop the key question that, if answered, would eliminate or ameliorate its difficulties. The question generally begins with "how can" or "how should," and it articulates the goal to be achieved in that problem area and the constraints that are preventing that goal from being achieved. These questions are called your issue statements.

4. Synthesize the issue statements into an overall problem statement. The problem statement is written in the same question format as the issue statements. It contains all of the interrelated aspects of the problem. You now have a problem definition—your problem statement.

What makes the steps difficult to implement in practice is related primarily to having the "never assume" mindset. This is what takes discipline and hard work. When faced with a problem, we implicitly start making assumptions about the problem, its root causes, and its solutions without realizing it. This is what is hard to change—the discipline of our thought process to never assume. In his book called *Thinking Fast and Slow*, Daniel Kahneman, the Nobel prize winning economist, describes jumping to solutions while making implicit assumptions, and drawing incorrect inferences because of this, as fast thinking.[2] The advantage of fast thinking is it reduces the cognitive load of solving problems. The drawback is that it will lead to solving the wrong problem, resulting in suboptimal solutions that don't solve the problem.

The "never assume" mindset requires that you stop making assumptions when defining the problem. You need to step outside of yourself as if you are an external, unbiased consultant viewing the situation in a fair, impartial manner. You set aside your biases and your preferences, and you always look in the mirror and ask yourself if you are part of the problem. And as you listen and watch for difficulties, you sort out facts from opinions. This deliberate approach is what Kahneman calls slow thinking. It is hard to accomplish because it increases the cognitive workload required to solve problems as you explicitly engage in information gathering and analysis. But, we posit that by practicing the core elements of problem definition of the Problem-Solving Method, you learn how to think slow and fast simultaneously. The "never assume" thought process becomes automatic. Like any other skill, it takes practice.

The other aspect of this approach to defining the problem that takes practice is writing the issue statements for the problem areas. Crafting issue statements is a higher order cognitive skill, as it requires synthesis and integration. Writing issue statements requires that you review the difficulties to discern the key issue in each problem area that needs resolution. If that key issue written in the form of a question is answered, then the difficulties in the problem area would either disappear or be alleviated. The set of issue statements define the interrelated components that comprise the problem.

With experience, you will rarely write out the issue statements or the problem statement. But, you will have inculcated in your brain the discipline of framing action-oriented "how can we" questions across the problem areas that invite action and do not have solutions embedded in them. When working with a team in an organization to solve a problem, the team should work collaboratively to ensure that all come to the same definition of the problem. Develop the problem areas, and come to an agreement on the key issue for each problem area. The issue statements can then be synthesized and integrated into the overall problem statement.

The other key strength of the Problem-Solving Method—engaging stakeholders—is useful not just for interacting with them to identify the difficulties in the situation. Through doing a thorough stakeholder analysis, you understand the situation from the multitude of points of view that exist in the organization. This understanding helps you develop a strategy for maximizing the probability that your final set of recommendations will be accepted and implemented.

In some cases, acceptance of the recommendations requires a formal vote of a decision-making body in the organization. In other cases, it requires consensus, but not a formal vote. Regardless, you need to develop a deliberate strategy for how you will get the "deciders" to say yes. But, it's more than focusing on just the stakeholders who are the "deciders." You need to ensure that any stakeholders who will be affected by the recommendations, and any who will be responsible for implementing the recommendations, are also on board. Thus, throughout the entire problem-solving process, you need to continuously keep the stakeholders' views in mind. For some, it means keeping them apprised of your work as you conduct your research and develop findings. For others, it means thinking through how they might react to your recommendations, and working through any opposition that may arise. By the time you are making your final presentation of your work and your recommended course of action, there should be no surprises. Your audience should not be surprised about what they are hearing from you, and you should not be surprised by unanticipated pushback or objections from them. Know your stakeholders.

In the remainder of this chapter, we compare and contrast the Problem-Solving Method in this field manual to Lean and Design Thinking, two of the most widely used methodologies in healthcare organizations.

LEAN

■ OVERVIEW OF LEAN

The Lean problem-solving methodology grew out of the auto manufacturing management philosophies and practices of continuous improvement at Toyota, called the Toyota Production System.[3] The mindset of Lean is to drive waste out of the organization's processes. It requires: (a) defining what is meant by value in a process; (b) engaging in value stream mapping of processes to eliminate non-value added steps; (c) striving for uniform continuous process flow; (d) "pulling" demand through the process; and (e) engaging in continuous improvement to develop and sustain incremental improvements in the process.[4]

Thus, Lean is a methodology designed to study processes in a system with a goal of incremental improvement to make them better. Lean relies on a variety of tools of quality in its repertoire of process improvement; for example, brainstorming, Pareto analysis, cause/effect diagrams (often called fishbone diagrams), 5 Whys root cause analysis, force field analysis, and A3 Problem-Solving Story visualization.[5]

Figure 3.1 shows the typical components of the A3 Problem-Solving Story visualization used in Lean. The A3 has four steps that are in the Plan phase, including: (a) documenting the background and context of the problem; (b) describing the current situation, in which the problem is stated and the process is mapped; (c) setting goals and targets; and (d) engaging in 5 Whys root cause analysis to identify the real problem. An additional three steps are in the Do, Check, Act phase, including: (a) identifying possible solutions; (b) implementing the actions and assigning accountability for implementation; and (c) monitoring results.

The problem-solving as described by the A3 is focused on processes internal to the organization. This impacts the structure of the problem statement. In Lean, the problem statement format is to state a fact that focuses on the symptom of what is wrong in the process under study (e.g., the patient is late to appointments). And, although the

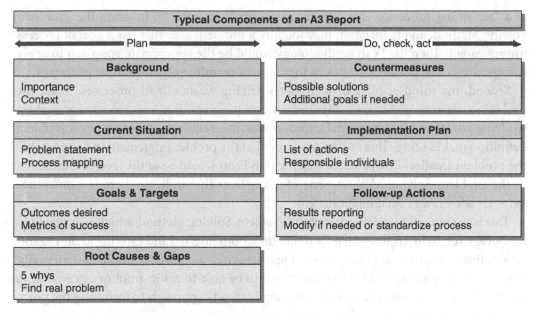

FIGURE 3.1 Typical components of a Lean A3 report.

problem statement should not assign a root cause or blame and should not include a solution, it is to be limited to one problem.[6]

Lean methods require a Lean culture in which staff learn and internalize three key elements of Lean: (a) standard work processes; (b) user-friendly processes; and (c) unobstructed throughput in the process.[7] Staff engagement in Lean often focuses on participation in Kaizen events. During these events, representative staff who work in the process help describe the current process and design an improved process that eliminates non-value–added activities.

In summary, Lean is a problem-solving methodology tailored for incremental change in processes. The value-stream map of the process is used to identify non-value–added steps in the process, from the viewpoint of the customer. The goal is to have continuous process flow or throughput. Staff involvement occurs in dedicated problem-solving events, called Kaizen events, to engage in process mapping and process redesign. Finally, it relies on a variety of analytic tools of quality improvement.

■ COMPARISON OF LEAN AND THE PROBLEM-SOLVING METHOD

As a problem-solving methodology, Lean shares similar terminology and steps with the Problem-Solving Method. This is to be expected, as they are both problem-solving approaches. But there are differences between Lean and the Problem-Solving Method.

First is the purpose of the method. The Lean methodology focuses on internal processes for incremental improvement. However, there are many problems in organizations that are not process problems. The Problem-Solving Method is a more general approach to problem-solving that is agnostic as to problem type. It can be thought of as a "reasoning processor" for organizational problem-solving. In using the Problem-Solving Method, an organization may identify a problem area that has a goal of process improvement. Then the Lean methodology would be the appropriate approach to apply specifically to that problem area as its focus is to streamline organizational processes.

Second, the mindset of Lean focuses on driving waste out of processes. Thus, the problem statement is narrowly focused on one problem. Because Lean is focused on studying processes for incremental improvement, this requirement for a narrow problem definition makes sense. This means, however, that the problem statement in Lean "makes the problem smaller." The problem statement in Lean would be at the level of a difficulty in the Problem-Solving Method—one of many facts that indicate there is a difference between what is and what ought to be.

This is in contrast to the mindset of the Problem-Solving Method, which is designed to encourage you to listen and watch for difficulties, both internal and external to the organization. Internally, there are many types of problems beyond process problems. Externally, you need to pay attention to the environment to be able to get in front of or respond to changes in your market. The Problem-Solving Method's approach to formulate the problem statement is to recognize that many organizational problems are interrelated "messes" of difficulties. The challenge in solving messy problems is figuring out how to chunk the mess up into manageable pieces—problem areas—that are as independent of each other as possible. Then, the issue statements identify the key goal-oriented questions that invite action, and that need to be answered to solve the problem. Thus, the problem statement in the Problem-Solving Method is designed to "make the problem bigger."

The other major difference between Lean and the Problem-Solving Method is the role of stakeholders in the methodology. In Lean, the customer viewpoint focuses on the value stream map of the process. Staff involvement focuses on mapping and improving processes to eliminate non-value–added activity. Thus, stakeholder involvement focuses on value-stream mapping of processes, not gaining stakeholder perspectives more broadly defined.

The Problem-Solving Method, on the other hand, has as a core principle to understand your stakeholders at a much more expansive level than Lean. The Define phase of the Method requires a stakeholder analysis, the Study phase includes a "hard stop" review step to circle back with key stakeholders, and the Act phase requires a communication strategy that focuses on how to tailor your message to stakeholders to maximize the probability of acceptance.

There are many quality tools used in Lean that are clearly relevant in many of the Problem-Solving Method's steps. For example, in the first step of the Study phase, tools such as brainstorming, fishbone diagrams, and 5 Whys root cause analysis can be helpful to generate root causes and alternative solutions. Analyzing data using Pareto analysis can help identify actual root causes when studying the problem. Force field analysis can be used to identify the forces pro and con for alternative solutions. And an A3 visualization can be used to summarize on one page a project that has been completed using the Problem-Solving Method. Thus, although the underlying philosophy and principles are different between Lean and the Problem-Solving Method, there are many tools of Lean that are complementary and useful to use in a number of steps in the Problem-Solving Method.

In summary, the Problem-Solving Method and Lean are both problem-solving methodologies. And, in fact, many of the steps look similar. However, the purpose and mindset of the methods are different. Lean is focused on processes, while the Problem-Solving Method is focused on broader organizational and management problems. As a result, the problem statement of Lean is narrowly focused on the symptom that indicates there is something wrong in the process. The problem statement of the Problem-Solving Method is the comprehensive set of key issues that must be resolved across the problem areas to correct a messy problem. To resolve the organizational problems, engaging stakeholders across all phases of the problem-solving process is a core component of the Problem-Solving Method, while in Lean, their involvement tends to be focused on mapping current and improved processes. Both methods are valuable, but their intended use is very different.

DESIGN THINKING AND HUMAN CENTERED DESIGN

In contrast to Lean, which focuses on incremental improvements in processes to remove non-value–added steps, Design Thinking and Human Centered Design are methods that are well suited for service or product design problems that are very hard to define, understand, and/or for which there is not a solution already developed. Design Thinking and Human-Centered Design are applicable when transformational change is needed, as incremental change has not worked. There are more similarities between the Problem-Solving Method and Design Thinking and Human-Centered Design compared to the Problem-Solving Method with Lean.

Before comparing and contrasting the Problem-Solving Method to Design methods, you can see that, similar to Lean, the Design methods focus on process, service, and product design, not broader organizational messy problems. It is interesting to note that in 1964, a seminal book on design, called *Notes on the Synthesis of Form,* was written by an architect called Christopher Alexander.[8] His book focused on more complex design problems, ones that have seemingly insoluble levels of complexity, for example, designing a complete environment for a million people. His design process for trying to make the design requirements problem tractable is conceptually identical to the Problem-Solving Method's approach of identifying difficulties and grouping them into problem areas.

Alexander describes a process in which all design requirements are listed. The list is too comprehensive to design for each of the requirements individually. Therefore, the next step he describes is to identify the subsets of requirements that positively interact with each other and group them. Once all the design requirements are grouped, there should be minimal interaction with the design requirements between groups. This greatly reduces the complexity of the design problem because it enables you to focus on designing for the tightly linked requirements within each group independent of the design requirements for the other groups. His approach reduces an intractable messy design process into a more conceptually compact, solvable design problem. This is exactly the rationale and approach used in the Problem-Solving Method for difficulties and problem area groupings.

■ DESIGN THINKING

Design thinking focuses on approaches for a deep understanding of end-user needs when designing services and products. There are a number of processes or models that are in use today. One model is the Double Diamond process coined by the British Design Council in 2004. Their model articulates four phases: Discover, Define, Develop, Deliver.[9] As shown in Figure 3.2, the key principles in their model of Design Thinking are related to engaging in cycles of divergent and convergent thinking to understand the desirability, viability, and feasibility of solutions that are created to solve a design problem. Each diamond represents a divergent-convergent cycle. The first cycle focuses on divergent thinking when engaging with end users to study the problem, and then converges on a problem definition and design brief. The next wave of divergent thinking focuses on iterative development of prototypes to learn which designs fail and which ones work in order to drive to a deliverable solution.

As described in Chapter 1, "The Problem Is Not Always What It Seems," the Problem-Solving Method has this similar double diamond wave of two cycles of divergent and convergent thinking. As shown in Figure 3.3, the first wave of divergent-convergent thinking focuses on defining the problem, while the second wave addresses arriving at a set of recommendations after studying the problem. Both methods also have as a core principle communicating with affected parties. In Design Thinking, the focus is on the end user who will be using a new product or process. In the Problem-Solving Method, the focus is all stakeholders who are touched by the problem in some way.

■ HUMAN-CENTERED DESIGN

Human-Centered Design in its modern terminology and thought, was coined by Mike Cooley in 1989 in his book *Human-Centered Systems*.[10] This approach is aligned with

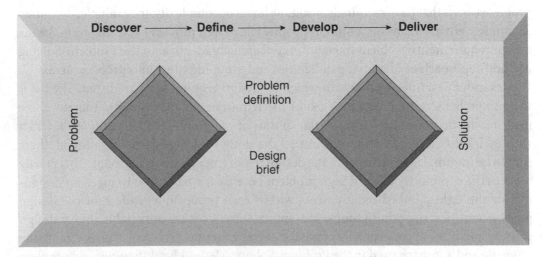

FIGURE 3.2 The "Double Diamond" of Design Thinking.

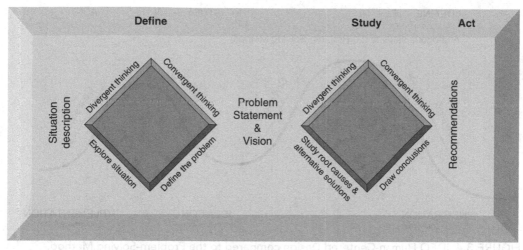

FIGURE 3.3 The "Double Diamond" of the Problem-Solving Method.

Design Thinking, although it more specifically articulates the steps and tools that are helpful to incorporate the user in solving problems and developing new approaches. In contrast to Design Thinking, the emphasis is more on the desirability equation in the design process. It was initially popular throughout technology and product companies to create new products with the "user" or human in mind throughout the entire process. In fact, the International Organization for Standardization (ISO), adopted elements in some of the standards and recommendations as well as the following definition of Human-Centered Design:

> *Human-centred design is an approach to interactive systems development that aims to make systems usable and useful by focusing on the users, their needs and requirements, and by applying human factors/ergonomics, and usability knowledge and techniques. This approach enhances effectiveness and efficiency, improves human well-being, user satisfaction, accessibility and sustainability; and counteracts possible adverse effects of use on human health, safety and performance.*[11]

The concept was taken further to products and services by the Founder of IDEO, Stanford Professor David Kelley. This organization and the methods and tools created have become popular throughout various industries. IDEO now serves as a consultancy firm and a teacher of the IDEO Design process. Many innovation centers throughout healthcare have deployed the techniques and tools developed by IDEO.[12]

A key similarity between Human-Centered Design and the Problem-Solving Method is the focus on understanding and involving the affected stakeholders in defining, studying and developing solutions to solve the key issues and problems. Both methods start with visiting with the stakeholders to make the problem "bigger" and engaging in divergent thinking to further understand the layers of the problem and identify difficulties. More information on the Human-Centered Design process as outlined by IDEO and its relationship to the Problem-Solving Method is highlighted in the following.

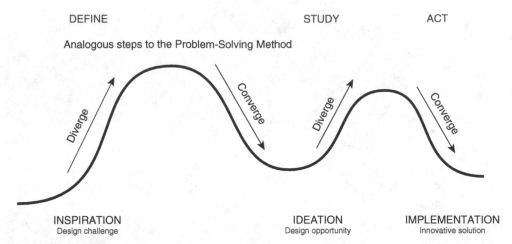

FIGURE 3.4 IDEO Human-Centered Design compared to the Problem-Solving Method.

IDEO Design Kit

In 2009, after almost a decade of increasing popularity of using Design Thinking and Human-Centered Design, IDEO sought to bring the method and tools to a greater audience. They created the IDEO Design Kit,[13] which is widely used throughout service and product design communities and innovation centers. The Design Kit describes Human-Centered Design in divergent and convergent thinking across three phases of Inspiration, Ideation, and Implementation as seen in Figure 3.4. The steps conducted in these phases are very similar to the Problem-Solving Method's three phases of Define, Study, Act.

Inspiration—Define

The inspiration phase in IDEO's Design Kit provides tools and methods to open up the stakeholder to provide information on their current situation. The intent is to acquire empathy for your customer, to see the world from their perspective, and leave behind your own biases. Many design projects purposely stay in this phase for quite some time in order to fully ensure they are uncovering articulated and unarticulated needs, or what we would call in the Problem-Solving Method, the difficulties and possible root causes. The tools used include observations, interviews, immersion, and illustration to name a few. Any problem solver using the Problem-Solving Method, particularly a novice or an expert experiencing a very complex problem could benefit from adopting the tools suggested to better understand stakeholders and the problem.

Ideation—Define and Study

Once the designer has acquired an empathetic understanding of the problem, they analyze and synthesize the information into themes. This is similar to the process of creating the stakeholder analysis and problem areas. Additionally, the designer will create opportunity statements that often begin with "How might we...." These statements, however, are a bit different than issue statements. This is where the design process and the Problem-Solving Method start to differ. Designers will create questions that will drive to the creation of a concept and then prototype it to acquire additional empathy and understanding of customer needs. In the Problem-Solving Method, the issue statements are more open ended, allowing for multiple alternatives to be listed/explored. The criteria developed will encompass many factors that will include stakeholder acceptability, although they also encompass organizational feasibility and viability alongside stakeholder acceptance. The criteria in the Problem-Solving Method will include more system elements such as efficiencies, quality outcomes, financial viability, and sustainability, for example. At some point in the ideation phase of IDEO, there is a decision to prototype one main idea to learn, iterate, and develop a solution. In the Problem-Solving Method, you typically are not building a prototype. You are exploring all options through multiple angles of research. This is not to say that you couldn't build a prototype to rule in or out one alternative, although this would be one factor to consider in deciding which alternative(s) to select, not the main factor.

Implementation —Act

Once a prototype is designed in the Ideation Phase, the designer and team start the prototype and begin to test for desirability, feasibility, and viability. As this is tested, the team may iterate to create a better design. When the signs are there, the team then moves to pilot and then scale. Stakeholders are involved in the process and feedback throughout the iterations. This is similar to the Problem-Solving Method, in that stakeholders should be brought along and are providing feedback throughout all of its phases to facilitate their understanding of the options and alternatives so they are not surprised at the end.

■ COMPLEMENTS, NOT COMPETITORS

Design Thinking, Human-Centered Design and the Problem-Solving Method have a great deal in common. They all require waves of divergent and convergent thinking, and they all require active stakeholder involvement, with empathy and listening a core part of learning from them to inform what the problem is and what the stakeholders need for its resolution. In addition, Human-Centered Design, particularly the IDEO Design Kit, provides those using the Problem-Solving Method with tools to dive deep into stakeholder needs when defining the problem, testing alternatives, and presenting recommendations for acceptance. In the final analysis, these two problem-solving frameworks are not separate or in competition with each other. Each has its role depending on the problem focus, and the Problem-Solving Method can tap into tools and elements from Design Thinking and Human-Centered Design to better engage with stakeholders.

COMPARISON SUMMARY

Table 3.1 provides a comparison of the three problem-solving methodologies.

TABLE 3.1 Comparison of Problem-Solving Methods

	PROBLEM-SOLVING METHOD	LEAN	DESIGN THINKING/ HUMAN-CENTERED DESIGN
Problem Focus	"Messy" organizational problem	Incremental process improvements	Innovative service, product, or process design
Stakeholder Involvement	Extensive throughout the process	Focus on customer process requirements and staff Kaisen events	Extensive throughout the process, focused on the end-user
Define the Problem	Difficulties and problem areas; issue statements and problem statement	Focus on one "problem," equivalent to the definition of a difficulty	Elicit customer requirements from end users, with many useful tools, design brief
Study the Problem	Generalized method that benefits from specific tools depending on the problem area	Tools of quality, with many useful analytic methods for root cause analysis and problem study	Multiple iterations of prototype solutions in collaboration with stakeholders
Act on the Problem	Develop set of integrated recommendations across all problem areas	Implement process improvements that reduce non-value–added steps	Hone in on and iterate prototype to determine plan to implement to scale

Of the three methods, the Problem-Solving Method has the broadest focus, as it is designed to identify and solve organizational level problems with many interrelated problem areas. This is in contrast to Lean and Design Thinking, which are focused on more specific targets, namely incremental process improvement (Lean) or innovative processes, products, or services design (Design Thinking). When using the Problem-Solving Method, there will be times when a problem area will require process improvement or broader process, product, or service innovation. In these situations, it is clearly useful to apply the specific methods and tools of Lean or Design Thinking to those problem areas.

Of the three methods, the Problem-Solving Method and Design Thinking have the most comprehensive approaches for engaging stakeholders in the process. In addition, the tools used in Design Thinking that engage stakeholders in problem definition can be useful for use in the problem-definition phase of the Problem-Solving Method.

Turning to problem definition, the goal of the Problem-Solving Method is to capture all aspects of the problem through identifying difficulties and grouping them into problem areas, followed by writing issue statements and the problem statement. Lean's approach is to narrow in on one problem definition of an organizational process, which in the Problem-Solving Method would be one difficulty of many that may need resolution. Design Thinking's goal is to elicit the end-user requirements to identify the design challenge.

In problem study, Lean uses many tools of quality, such as fishbone diagrams and 5 Whys, that are particularly useful in the Problem-Solving Method when engaging in root cause analysis and data analysis. Thus, this is an area in which the Problem-Solving Method can draw upon Lean tools. Finally in the act phase, the Problem-Solving Method requires an integrated set of recommendations across all the areas that solve the problem as defined. Lean results in process improvements that reduce non-value–added steps, and Design Thinking ends with an innovative product, process, or service that can be brought to scale.

Of the three methods, the Problem-Solving Method is agnostic as to the type of problem being faced, and can be thought of as a "logic processor" to apply in any situation when engaging in organizational problem-solving. As it is applied, there are tools from the other two methods that will be useful. And, depending on the problem areas uncovered, there will be situations in which either the entire Lean or Design Thinking approach should be used as a tailored approach in those problem areas, because the identified issue involves either incremental process improvement (Lean) or fundamental process, service, or product redesign (Design Thinking).

In summary, all of the problem-solving methods highlighted in this chapter are useful. You should get to know all of them, and gain experience in recognizing what type of problem you are facing to pull from the appropriate method or tools to solve the problem.

REFERENCES

1. Ackoff RL. *Redesigning the future: a systems approach to societal problems*. New York, NY: John Wiley & Sons; 1974.
2. Kahneman D. *Thinking fast and slow*. New York, NY: Farrar, Straus, and Giroux; 2011.
3. Liker J. *The Toyota way: 14 management principles from the world's greatest manufacturer*. New York, NY: McGraw-Hill; 2004.
4. Womack JP, Jones DT. *Lean thinking: banish waste and create wealth in your corporation*. New York, NY: Free Press; 2003.
5. Iuga MV, Rosca LI. *Comparison of problem solving tools in Lean organizations*. MATEC Web of Conferences; 2017.
6. McMahon T. *Problem solving starts with defining the problem* [blog post]. 2015. http://www.aleanjourney .com/2015/07/problem-solving-starts-with-defining.html
7. Zidel TG. *Lean done right: achieve and maintain reform in your healthcare organization*. Chicago, IL: Health Administration Press; 2012.
8. Alexander C. *Notes on the synthesis of form*. Cambridge, MA: Harvard University Press; 1973. (Original work published in 1964).
9. Design Council. *What is the framework for innovation? Design council's evolved double diamond*. [News and opinions]. 2019. https://www.designcouncil.org.uk/news-opinion/what-framework-innovation-design -councils-evolved-double-diamond
10. Cooley M. (1989). Human-centred systems. In: *The Springer series on artificial intelligence and society*. New York, NY: Springer Link; 1989:133–143.
11. ISO. *Ergonomics of human-system interaction—Part 210: Human-centred design for interactive systems*. 2019. https://www.iso.org/obp/ui/#iso:std:iso:9241:-210:ed-2:v1:en
12. IDEO. *How we work*. 2019. https://www.ideo.com/about
13. IDEO. *Design kit: the human centered design tool kit*. 2019. https://www.ideo.com/post/design-kit

CHAPTER 4

MANAGEMENT AND LEADERSHIP COMPETENCIES OF THE PROBLEM-SOLVING METHOD

INTRODUCTION

People who do well in senior management positions are those who are very good at problem-solving and issue resolution, particularly when they lack specific knowledge or information. I'd try to focus on getting my students to identify the problem and how to solve it, not whether they could recite some particular theory or model. Educators should not allow students to merely parrot back memorized content, but should test the students' skill at problem-solving. While content changes over time, good problem-solving never goes out of date. [1(p241)]

—Jerry Jurgensen, former CEO of Nationwide

DEVELOPING YOUR PROBLEM-SOLVING COMPETENCIES

Problem-solving is more than just solving problems. To be a good problem solver, you also need to know how to listen, how to communicate, how to "read" an organization, how to have confidence in yourself and your abilities, and how to think critically, among many other skills. Thus, as you develop your capabilities in mastering the Problem-Solving Method, you develop these other competencies, which are essential managerial and leadership competencies. This chapter describes the competencies that you will develop through mastering the Problem-Solving Method. For those of you who want to jump right in to practicing the Problem-Solving Method, we recommend that you first practice the Method in Parts II, III, and IV of the text, and come back to this chapter later.

■ SKILLS VERSUS COMPETENCIES

As teachers, we have found that our healthcare management students highly value the coursework that develops their mastery of content and skills in the functional areas of business, such as operations, strategy, finance, and data analytics. These skills are important and necessary, but not sufficient, for you to be viewed as highly desirable by employers. Employers expect that you will also be competent in critical thinking, problem-solving, judgment and decision-making, communicating, and teamwork.

There is a difference between skills and competencies. The difference is that competencies are more than skills; competencies additionally include abilities, behaviors, and psychosocial resources to meet complex demands.[2]

As described in this chapter, these competencies being sought by employers are generally referred to as "soft skills," while the functional business content areas, also sought by employers, are referred to as "hard skills." This is an unfortunate misnomer, because "the soft stuff is actually the hard stuff."[3(p225)] Thus, while developing yourself to have a successful career, it is just as important to develop your management and leadership competencies as it is your foundational knowledge of functional areas of business. The later sections of this chapter describe how the Problem-Solving Method helps you develop these "soft skill" management and leadership competencies. For those of you who are experienced managers but new to healthcare management, an overview of the leadership competencies described in this chapter are specific to healthcare, developed by the National Center for Healthcare Leadership.

Even with limited real-world experience, the Problem-Solving Method can help you develop management and leadership competencies in your coursework, your summer residency or internship, your capstone projects, your post-graduate fellowship and early in your professional career. Through using the Problem-Solving Method, you can start to make an impact in healthcare right away, starting in graduate school. In our years in teaching problem-solving, it has been typical for the student project recommendations to be implemented by the host organization. And, there are generally a few projects every year in which the project recommendations were projected to save the organization hundreds of thousands of dollars, and sometimes more.

■ PROBLEM-SOLVING FOR REAL-WORLD PROJECTS

There are two aspects to developing your problem-solving skills using the Problem-Solving Method: (a) mastering the steps and substeps of the Define, Study, and Act phases; and (b) using the method to solve an actual management problem in an organization. To master the steps, you should work through all of the activities in Parts II, III, and IV of the text, using The Spinal Frontier case and additional cases we have provided in Part V. To master using the Problem-Solving Method in real-life projects, we recommend the following approach.

Problem-Solving Project Milestones

In real-world projects in organizations, you want to demonstrate that you know how to approach your project work, as opposed to having to rely on your preceptor or boss to give you constant detailed step-by-step directions on what you need to do next. The structure of the Problem-Solving Method provides a logical framework with natural built-in deliverables to, and touchpoints with, your preceptor, mentor, or boss as you work on your project. You will come prepared to your weekly or regularly scheduled meetings with your preceptor with written deliverables to discuss.

Thus, you will take the initiative to keep the project moving forward, rather than passively waiting for your preceptor to tell you what to do. This helps you have confidence in taking initiative by using a logical framework for how to approach your project work, versus not knowing where to start or what to do. You will know what work approach to propose, helping build trust of others about your capabilities early in your school and internship projects and your career.

Your meetings with your preceptors will focus on feedback and guidance on your work. Examples of meeting touchpoints and deliverables include:

Deliverable and Touchpoint #1: Come to agreement on your written situation description and scope of work, and a proposed list of stakeholders to interview.

Deliverable and Touchpoint #2: Review your written difficulties, problem areas, issue statement, problem statement, and vision for the future. Determine if all the problem areas can be addressed in the project's time frame, and if not, revise the scope.

Deliverable and Touchpoint #3: For each problem area, review your written possible root causes, potential alternative solutions, and decision criteria for comparing alternatives. Review your interview guide and research plan.

Deliverable and Touchpoint #4: Midway in your research, provide a written summary of what you have learned, and what you are concluding to date around your alternative solutions under consideration, and the selection criteria you will use to determine what to recommend.

Deliverable and Touchpoint #5: A written summary of your research, your conclusions, your recommendations, and your key milestones.

Deliverable and Touchpoint #6: A draft of your final presentation and a draft of your final written report.

Deliverable and Touchpoint #7: Your final presentation and final report.

Problem-Solving and Career Milestones

In a post-graduate fellowship or in your first post-graduate position, you will generally be working under a preceptor's direction, or with a project manager. In many cases, you will be part of a team working on a much larger scope project. In these situations, you will rarely be responsible for conducting all steps of the Problem-Solving Method.

As you work with the team, you will typically be assigned the role of information collector, observer, data analyst, and project manager, not the synthesizer of the information or the decision-maker. At this stage of your career, you will most likely be asked to perform organizing and information-gathering activities. Organizing activities include organizing meetings; developing agendas for meetings; ensuring the meeting room is set up correctly; taking thorough, complete and accurate minutes of meetings; identifying post-meeting action items; and facilitating the team's processes for getting its work accomplished.

Information-gathering activities will typically entail determining relevant data to be collected to identify and study a problem, developing a plan to collect it efficiently and effectively, interviewing stakeholders and experts, analyzing data, and summarizing the data in a meaningful way. As a fellow, you should actively seek out opportunities and volunteer to collect information, organize it, and present it to your team in a meaningful way.

As you gain experience, you will be asked not just to collect and organize information, but to synthesize the information to make judgments about it. Can you identify the key issues in a situation? Can you identify potential solutions and related decision criteria? Given the data collected, can you draw relevant, logical, and well-reasoned conclusions, and express them in a way that makes sense to the team? Can you develop recommendations based on those conclusions?

Finally, as you demonstrate your capabilities in making sound judgments, you will progress to making decisions. At this stage, you are viewed as an opinion leader by your colleagues, team members, supervisors, managers, and executives. You will be responsible for overseeing all phases of the Problem-Solving Method, and will be seen as the person who has the standing in the organization to facilitate getting consensus and approval from key stakeholders to move the recommendations forward.

In addition to the progression of skills described, the Problem-Solving Method facilitates your development of management and leadership competencies as described in the following.

MANAGEMENT SOFT SKILLS

■ HARD SKILLS VERSUS SOFT SKILLS

The core courses of management studies curricula have tended to focus on foundational business functions that are referred to as the "hard skills"—for example, finance, strategy, analytics, operations, accounting, marketing, and so forth. These topics have been defined or described as content expertise,[3] and "the technical or administrative procedures that can be quantified and measured."[4(p35)] But beginning in the early 2000s, there was increasing criticism that management curricula were losing relevancy.[5] For example, in the Master of Business Administration (MBA) literature, Mintzberg, in his book *Managers not MBAs*, argued that management is not a compilation of business functions, and that MBA curricula were failing to provide education in the art and practice of management.[6]

In response to the criticism of MBA program curricula, there has been an increasing emphasis on what are called the "soft skills." These are essential competencies expected by employers for success in the workplace over and above the "hard skills." Soft skills have been defined in many different ways. Interpersonal skills, teamwork, responsibility, emotional intelligence, critical thinking, and social skills are examples of what is captured by the term "soft skills."[3,7] A systematic review by Fisher of published articles, online MBA surveys, and other unpublished literature identified nineteen soft competencies, of which only six were judged by the study results as indicating that employers said were met.[5] These nineteen competencies are shown in Table 4.1, organized by whether they were deemed as met or not met by employers.

The study found that the top three essential soft competencies which were deemed as not being met by employers were work experience, critical thinking, and problem-solving.

TABLE 4.1 Nineteen Soft Competencies Judged as Met/Not Met by Employers

SOFT COMPETENCIES NOT MET	SOFT COMPETENCIES MET
Apply Work Experience	Teamwork
Critical Thinking Skills	Entrepreneurial Spirit
Problem-Solving	Display Integrity
Communication (Write and Speak Effectively)	Ethics (Honesty)
Leadership	Understand Difficulty in Starting a Business
Community Involvement (Contribute Positively)	Understand Business Goals and Objectives
Understand Importance of Customer in Business	
Listening	
Self-Accountability and Self-Awareness	
Professionalism	
Collaborate and Network	
Keeping up With Changing Technologies	
Apply Accounting Financial Skills (Plan and Budget)	

Source: From Fisher RD. A triangulation assessment: The value of an MBA degree, an evidenced-based management (EBMGT) systematic review (SR). *Academy of Educational Leadership Journal.* 2019;23(1):1–14.

The article cited several definitions of critical thinking, including: (a) being able to "think on your feet," and analyze what is going on in the organization[8]; (b) finding creative solutions to complex problems[9]; and (c) being able to differentiate facts from opinions, gather evidence, and develop and persuasively articulate logical and coherent arguments.[10] Problem-solving was described in the context that problems cross organizational boundaries, and that successful problem-solving requires being able to span these boundaries.[11]

The Problem-Solving Method clearly addresses these top three unmet competencies. As described in the initial section of this chapter, work experience is facilitated by providing an approach to help novice students and recent graduates who have limited experience successfully solve real-world problems in organizations. And the Problem-Solving Method clearly supports developing problem-solving skills.

In critical-thinking skills development, the Define phase teaches you how to identify difficulties, separate fact from opinion, group difficulties into problem areas, and identify the key issues. This supports your ability to "think on your feet" and understand what is going on in the organization.

In the Study phase, divergent thinking encourages generating and studying novel solutions. The structure of this phase also supports your ability to demonstrate the flow of your logic from the problem statement through to your findings, conclusions, and recommendations. Finally, the Act phase includes a communication strategy to develop your persuasion abilities.

The Problem-Solving Method also supports other soft competencies listed in Table 4.1. For example, the stakeholder analysis develops your listening skills and understanding your customers. Learning how to call upon experts and internal and external colleagues when conducting research in the Study phase develops your networking skills. Developing and implementing a communication strategy develops your communication skills. And perhaps most importantly, the "never assume" mindset of the Problem-Solving Method helps you develop self-awareness.

■ ROLES AND RESPONSIBILITIES OF MANAGERS

Moving beyond discrete lists of soft skills, Mintzberg's 2013 book, *Simply Managing: What Managers Do—And Can Do Better,* describes the roles and responsibilities of managers.[12]

The day-to-day environment in which managers work rarely allows for uninterrupted, systematic, reflective time to solve problems. Instead, Mintzberg's research has documented that a manager's time and attention are fragmented, having to focus briefly on one situation before transitioning to another. Within this fragmented environment, they have to decide what action to take. In light of the fragmentation of time and attention, how does a manager problem solve without stepping away from their role or daily duties?

And when they take action, they have to be able to engage in both analysis and synthesis. Managers must chunk issues into component pieces for analysis, but then reconnect them through synthesis. Mintzberg refers to this as the Labyrinth of Decomposition. The manager must understand the big picture, and from that big picture has to decide on the series of actions to take. In deciding on a course of action, the manager often has limited or erroneous hard data available on which to support their decision-making about a course of action.

Mintzberg describes managing as working along three dimensions: managing information, actions, and people. A well-rounded manager balances among these three dimensions. In considering the parts of a managers role, Mintzberg describes the following dimensions that are at work simultaneously.

Managing Information

In managing information, managers are the nerve center for their area of responsibility. They gather information not just through talking, but viscerally through multiple modes of seeing, listening, and feeling.

When working in the Problem-Solving Method, the information dimension, or the manager nerve center, uncovers difficulties in multiple ways—a one sentence email, a passing conversation in the hallway, an organizational report—and it becomes second nature for managers to recognize them. Once identified, the manager needs to determine if the situation requires management attention for resolution given other pressing needs in the organization, and if so, what parts of the situation, how quickly, and by whom—the scope.

Taking Action

In taking action, managers engage both proactively and reactively. Proactively, they plan and budget, and they develop organizational capabilities to respond to situations through networking and delegation. Reactively, they respond to situations that affect the organization, relying on organizational capabilities they have proactively developed.

When working in the Problem-Solving Method, the action dimension is represented in developing the problem areas and identifying the issue statements and the problem statement. The difficulties are chunked into problem areas to support analysis. The key issue in each problem area is identified by asking the *action-oriented question* that needs to be addressed. The issue statements are then synthesized into an overall problem statement that articulates the big picture of the problem that needs resolution. Depending on the situation, this may take no more than a few minutes in the manager's head, or it may take an appointed team with dedicated time to define the problem.

Managing People

In managing people, managers determine staffing, they clarify roles and responsibilities, and they manage conflict and team building.

Within the Problem-Solving Method, depending on the situation and scope, the manager either takes on the problem themselves, or delegates the responsibility to explore and resolve the problem to a person or team who has been developed and mentored to solve organizational problems. As part of managing conflict, the stakeholder analysis supports understanding the situation from multiple perspectives to aid in identifying the list of difficulties and a range of alternative solutions and goals.

Across the three dimensions, there are additional leadership aspects that include developing an organizational vision (information), engaging in entrepreneurship and strategic planning and execution (action), and growing people through supporting, motivating, inspiring, developing, and mentoring them (people).

The Problem-Solving Method is a practice-enabled approach that supports the development of managerial soft skills. In addressing Mintzberg's roles of the manager, the Problem-Solving Method supports developing competencies across his three dimensions of management—information, action, and people. And, by modeling the "never assume" mindset and developing others in the organization to engage in effective problem-solving, the manager supports Mintzberg's fourth managerial competency of leadership in managing people—developing, mentoring, and supporting people in the organization to become effective problem solvers.

HEALTHCARE LEADERSHIP COMPETENCIES

■ NATIONAL CENTER FOR HEALTHCARE LEADERSHIP COMPETENCY MODEL©

Around the same time of growing concerns about the relevance of MBA curricula in the early 2000s, similar criticisms were being raised by academicians and practitioners about healthcare graduate management education. In response, the National Center for Healthcare Leadership (NCHL) embarked on an extensive study of healthcare administration professionals who are early in their careers to identify the leadership competencies they need to be successful.[13] NCHL developed its leadership competency model based on their extensive field research. The model supports professional development as well as the assessment of leadership competencies in professional graduate healthcare management programs. The NCHL Health Leadership Competency Model has been recently updated to version 3.0 based on its latest research.[14]

The NCHL Leadership Competency Model is an integrated set of competencies that describes what is expected for successful career progression as a healthcare leader. The model is comprised of 28 competencies across seven domains, four of which are action domains, and three of which are enabling domains. The four action domains include Boundary Spanning, Execution, Transformation, and Relations. These four domains are comprised of 21 competencies, which are required for leaders to successfully carry out their direct work. The remaining seven competencies are part of the three enabling domains of: (a) Personal, Organizational, and Professional Values; (b) Health Systems Awareness and Business Literacy; and (c) Self-Awareness and Self-Development. The competencies in these three domains support the ability to be effective in the competencies of the action domains.

Each competency has behavioral descriptions with several levels of proficiency described. The vast majority of the competencies are what would be considered to be "soft skills" in management literature. The full model, including the definitions and levels of the 28 competencies, can be requested at www.nchl.org/page?page=272.

Other health professions schools have also integrated "soft skills" in their curriculum. Schools of Public Health, for example, are now required as part of their accreditation standards to include and assess the foundational "soft competencies" of leadership, communication, interprofessional teamwork practice, and systems thinking.[15]

■ HEALTHCARE LEADERSHIP COMPETENCIES OF THE PROBLEM-SOLVING METHOD

Seventeen of the 28 NCHL competencies are addressed in one or more phases, steps, or substeps of the Problem-Solving Method. This section provides an overview of how the Problem-Solving Method maps to the NCHL competencies, shown in Table 4.2. (We have collapsed the Writing and Speaking Communication Skills competencies into one row in the table.)

Eleven of the NCHL competencies are developed across all three phases of the Problem-Solving Method, including Analytical Thinking, Change Leadership, Collaboration, Communication Skills (Writing and Speaking/Facilitating), Impact and Influence, Information Seeking, Innovation, Interpersonal Understanding, Organizational Awareness, and Self-Confidence. In addition, the Interpersonal Understanding competency is also addressed by the "never assume" mindset.

Two additional NCHL competencies are addressed by the "never assume" mindset. These are Self-Awareness and Values. In addition, the Self-Awareness competency is a key aspect in the Define phase.

The remaining four NCHL leadership competencies covered by the Problem-Solving Method—Collaboration, Process Improvement, and Strategic Orientation—occur in one or two phases each.

TABLE 4.2 Mapping the Problem-Solving Method to the National Center for Healthcare Leadership (NCHL) Competencies

	"NEVER ASSUME"	DEFINE	STUDY	ACT
Analytical Thinking		X	X	X
Change Leadership		X	X	X
Collaboration		X	X	X
Communication Skills*		X	X	X
Impact and Influence		X	X	X
Information Seeking		X	X	X
Initiative		X		
Innovation		X	X	X
Interpersonal Understanding	X	X	X	X
Organizational Awareness		X	X	X
Performance Measurement				X
Process and Quality Improvement			X	X
Self-Awareness	X	X		
Self-Confidence		X	X	X
Strategic Orientation		X		X
Values	X			

*This is two separate competencies: 1. Writing and 2. Speaking and Facilitating
Source: Data from the National Center for Healthcare Leadership.

A description of how the Problem-Solving Method addresses the competencies is given in the following.

Analytical Thinking

The Analytical Thinking competency is supported by teaching you to internalize a structured process that supports your ability to break a problem into its component pieces to accurately define it, understand the root cause drivers, research alternative solutions to arrive at well-reasoned conclusions, and provide a set of recommendations that resolves all the interrelated aspects of the problem as defined.

Change Leadership

Change Leadership is covered most fully in the Define phase and the Act phase. In the Define phase, you develop the ability to identify the need for change by utilizing the approach for defining problems—identifying difficulties, grouping them into problem areas, identifying the key issue that needs resolution in each problem area, and then synthesizing the issues into an overall problem statement. You also create a vision for the future that helps stakeholders understand what the organization will look like if the problem is successfully resolved. In the Act phase, Change Leadership occurs in the communication strategy step. In this step, you need to identify and implement a strategy for "getting to yes" for your recommended course of action. This requires an understanding of where resistance may lie, and how it can best be overcome.

Change Leadership also occurs in the Study phase, although it is more subtle. As you develop findings when you research the problem, you may come to the conclusion that a preferred solution of a powerful stakeholder is not a viable alternative. Or you may conclude from your findings that a solution vehemently opposed to by a powerful stakeholder is in fact the alternative that rises to the top for recommendation. If you want your recommendations be implemented in the Act phase, you need to determine when and how to deliver this message as soon as possible to the stakeholder, and other key stakeholders, to get their buy-in about your findings, what you are concluding based on these findings, and what the implications are for the best course of action for the organization.

Collaboration

The Problem Solving Method requires soliciting input from a wide range of people. You need to engage with people, actively seek their input, and genuinely appreciate it. There may be times they tell you things you don't want to hear. But that doesn't make their input less valuable.

In the Define phase, you seek input as you develop a description of the situation and conduct a stakeholder analysis.

In the Study phase, you seek input as you develop possible root causes and potential alternative solutions, and as you interact with experts, colleagues, and stakeholders when conducting your research.

In the Act phase, you actively solicit input as you communicate in multiple ways with key stakeholders. Another important aspect of collaboration occurs in your oral presentation. There may be parts of your presentation, for example, key recommendations, that were the idea of someone other than you. If that is the case, thank them and give them the credit publicly. It was their idea, so make it theirs.

Communication Skills

Writing, speaking, and facilitation are paramount across all of the phases. In the Define phase, your speaking and facilitation skills are developed through learning how to interact with key stakeholders to understand what is going on in a situation, and in engaging in guided conversations with a wide range of stakeholders as you complete a thorough stakeholder analysis. You develop your writing skills by learning how to write clear, crisp, and concise issue statements and problem statements that in totality capture all aspects of the problem. As you gain experience, you usually will not write out the issue statements, but will learn how to articulate them verbally in real time.

In the Study phase, facilitation skills, such as brainstorming, are key to developing a comprehensive set of possible root causes and potential alternative solutions. You also improve your ability to interview experts and colleagues, internal and external to the organization, as you gather findings while conducting your research. You also practice how to write persuasively through summarizing your findings, forming judgments based on them, and then synthesizing your work into an overall set of conclusions. Your writing should clearly articulate the logic trail of how you got from your findings to your conclusions.

Speaking skills are paramount in the Act phase. In the communication strategy step, you will almost always be making an oral presentation about your project in front of an audience of key stakeholders. The purpose of this presentation is to get the key stakeholders to say "yes." Thus, your presentation must be persuasive. You are typically also required to summarize your work in a written format that demonstrates your thought process in an engaging way that convinces the reader that you have arrived at a set of well-reasoned recommendations and action plan for the organization.

Impact and Influence

The focus of the stakeholder analysis on understanding the perceptions, goals, motivations, and interests of the key stakeholders; how they vary between the stakeholder groups; and how to develop a communications strategy to address these differing views, helps you develop your abilities in the Impact and Influence competency. In the Define phase, you learn how to conduct a stakeholder analysis to truly understand your stakeholders.

In the Study phase, you continue to assess their positions as you develop your findings and conclusions to determine how to engage them for input and feedback as you begin to think about how to gain buy-in for your conclusions and recommendations.

In the Act phase, you develop a well-thought out communications strategy that informs and persuades stakeholders through multiple approaches to gain support for your recommendations and action plan for the organization.

Information Seeking

The Information Seeking competency is a key competency mastered in the Problem-Solving Method. You should always be scanning for difficulties or opportunities in the organization (Define phase). It should become second nature to how you do your work. As difficulties are uncovered, you will follow up with people familiar with the situation to learn more, and based on what you learn, determine if the situation needs more study. If yes, you will engage in more in-depth fact finding through conducting a stakeholder analysis.

In the Study phase, you will engage in root cause analysis, alternative generation, and research, seeking out information from a variety of sources, including experts, colleagues, stakeholders, written reports, journal articles, and websites.

Finally, in the Act phase, you will seek understanding from stakeholders as you develop and implement a communications strategy.

Initiative

The Initiative competency involves identifying problems or opportunities and taking action proactively. Sometimes this action must be short-term, while other times it may be longer-term. And, in crisis situations, the action must happen immediately.

This competency is addressed in the Define phase of the Problem-Solving Method. In this phase, you identify a situation and difficulties that need attention, group the difficulties into problem areas, develop the issue statement for each problem area, and determine the priority order of the problem areas. Sometimes, a problem area needs immediate attention, while other times a problem area contains a long-term issue. As you gain experience, you will develop this action-oriented mindset as part of your automatic thought process to determine the timing and order of action. This approach also pertains to opportunities, not just problems.

Innovation

The Innovation competency addresses being able to help the organization in new and breakthrough ways. In the Define phase, the approach of the Problem-Solving Method supports framing the problem in a way that clarifies the complex, interrelated aspects of organizational problems. This approach is especially helpful when a team has become "stuck" in their work because there isn't agreement on what the problem is. The discipline of grouping difficulties into problem areas, and crafting issue and problem statements, helps reframe the problem to build agreement on what the problem is. You will be looked upon as an opinion leader in the organization as you develop the ability to "boil down" the mess of interrelated difficulties into a handful of problem areas, and articulate the key issue in each problem area that needs to be addressed.

In the Study phase, the idea generation in root causes and alternative solutions encourages engaging in divergent thinking to arrive at new ways of thinking about root cause drivers and developing novel alternatives. This is a step in which tools from Quality Improvement and Design Thinking can be used to support structured ways to drive innovative thinking. During your research, you will uncover best practices that are appropriate for your organization. In the Act phase, you need to determine how to adapt the best practices for successful implementation in your organization.

Interpersonal Understanding

Part of being an effective problem solver is being open to views and perspectives that are very different from your own, and actively seeking to understand people's goals and motivations. This is what is entailed in the Interpersonal Understanding competency. The "never assume" mindset, which requires that you understand yourself and understand your stakeholders, supports the development of this competency. The stakeholder analysis, the findings you develop in your research, and your communications strategy also require and reinforce your ability to look at the problem, its possible root causes, and its potential alternative solutions, from many different viewpoints.

Organizational Awareness

All organizations have their own unique cultures and traditions, which greatly affect how work gets done, how easy or hard change is, and who in the organization has decision-making authority. These aspects of organizations can be subtle, and it takes contextual experience to develop an understanding of the organization in which you are working.

Organizational Awareness entails understanding and using the formal and informal power structures in the organization, understanding the organization's culture, climate, history, and traditions and its impact on "how things get done," and understanding the values of the various stakeholder groups in the organization and using this knowledge to affect organizational change. You may have the best recommendations in the world, but if you lack organizational awareness, you might not be able to get them implemented.

In the Define phase, conducting a stakeholder analysis will help you gain deep insights into many aspects of organizational awareness. In the Study phase, aspects of organizational awareness are particularly important in developing decision criteria for judging alternative solutions. There may be alternatives that may just not be a good fit for the organization at this point in time for cultural or historical reasons. Cultures that are not accepting of innovation, for example, may not be ready for a revolutionary solution.

In the Act phase, organizational awareness is key to gaining acceptance of your recommendations. Sometimes, it may be stakeholders with informal authority that will have the power to prevent your recommendations from being approved. These are all issues you need to sort out as you conduct your stakeholder analysis so that you can develop a communication strategy to enhance your probability of successful implementation of your recommendations.

Performance Measurement

The Performance Measurement competency is relevant in the Implementation and Monitoring substep of the Act phase. This is the last substep of the Problem-Solving Method, and it entails being able to articulate what measures, metrics, and benchmarks should be tracked for each recommendation to ensure it is having its intended impact. You will also need to articulate how the data will be collected, who will monitor the metric, with what frequency, and what criteria will be used to determine if the recommendations have fixed the problem.

Process and Quality Improvement

As described in Chapter 3, the Study and Act phases of the Problem-Solving Method benefit from the use of tools from quality improvement methods such as Lean and Design Thinking. In the Study phase, identifying and studying root causes are facilitated by using process flow maps and cause and effect diagrams, for example. Design Thinking and Human-Centered Design tools can be used to generate and study alternatives.

In the Act phase, the use of Gantt charts supports the development and tracking of implementation plans for the recommendations. And, being able to benchmark to track performance is necessary to determine if the recommendations are working as intended.

Self-Awareness

To grow as a leader, you develop self-awareness by understanding your strengths and areas for improvement. And you need to be willing to accept feedback from others about how your behavior may be impacting them. Both the "never assume" mindset of knowing yourself and the Define phase help you develop self-awareness.

Knowing yourself requires that you identify your personal biases, and always ask yourself if you are part of the problem—is your management or leadership contributing to difficulties being faced in the situation? If yes, you need to be open and honest to the fact that you may need to change to improve organizational performance.

Self-Confidence

As discussed at the outset in this chapter, as a student or early careerist, it can seem daunting to be expected to know how to conduct a project in an organization. At the start of each academic year, the first year full-time MHA students at the University of Minnesota listen to the second year students describe their summer residency projects. The initial reaction of the first year students is sometimes fear—they wonder how they will be able to perform in this role when the time comes for their summer residency.

Learning the Problem-Solving Method will help you gain self-confidence in being able to perform in an organizational role. It does this in a number of ways. The logical structure of the phases, steps, and substeps provides you with a framework or approach for your project. You can proactively engage in your work, and use your meeting time with your preceptor or boss to discuss what you are discovering as you conduct your project. This enables you to engage with your preceptor or boss more like a mentor, rather than relying on them for detailed step-by-step instructions for how to carry out your work. This also facilitates their being able to have more time to share contextual knowledge about the organization or the healthcare industry relevant for your project.

Engaging with stakeholders and conducting research by reaching out to experts colleagues, and stakeholders improves your ability to ask thoughtful, probing questions. Analyzing difficulties and synthesizing them into problem areas and identifying the key issues increases your self-confidence in your higher order thinking skills. And developing a well-articulated story for an oral presentation, and presenting and defending your work in front of an audience of stakeholders, will improve your self-confidence in how to sell your ideas.

Values

The Values competency requires honesty and integrity. This is addressed in the "never assume" mindset that requires you to understand your stakeholders, and engage in cycles of divergent and convergent thinking. This facilitates your commitment to not jump prematurely to conclusions, but first and foremost focus on a full unbiased understanding of the problem. As you model this mindset, and mentor others in the Problem-Solving Method, the competency can grow from being a Personal Value to an Organizational Value.

PROBLEM-SOLVING IS NOT JUST SOLVING PROBLEMS

In summary, the Problem-Solving Method provides you with a logical, structured approach to identify, study, and solve organizational problems with a "never assume" mindset. As you practice the Problem-Solving Method, it will become the way you think without having to think about it.

But, as this chapter has described, it does more than that. In mastering the Problem-Solving Method, you will simultaneously be developing skills and competencies that will support developing your capabilities to become a manager and leader, regardless of your positional authority in the organization.

REFERENCES

1. Lewicki RJ. Jerry Jurgensen, Chief Executive Officer of Nationwide, on Mintzberg's Managers Not MBAs. *Acad Manag Learn Educ.* 2005;4(2):240–243. doi:10.5465/amle.2005.17268574
2. The Peak Performance Center. *Difference between competencies and skills.* 2019. http://thepeakperformancecenter.com/business/learning/course-design/learning-goals-objectives-outcomes/difference-between-competencies-and-skills
3. Parlamis J, Monno MJ. Getting to the CORE: putting an end to the term "soft skills." *J Manag Inq.* 2019;28(2):225–227. doi:10.1177/1056492618818023
4. Dixon J, Belnap C, Albrecht C, Lee K. The importance of soft skills. *Corporate Finance Review.* 2010;14(6):35–38.
5. Fisher RD. A triangulation assessment: the value of an MBA degree, an evidenced-based management (EBMGT) systematic review (SR). *Acad Educ Leadersh J.* 2019;23(1):1–14.
6. Mintzberg H. *Managers not MBAs: a hard look at the soft practice of managing and management development.* San Francisco, CA: Berrett-Koehler Publishers, Inc; 2004.
7. Robles MM. Executive perceptions of the top 10 soft skills needed in today's workplace. *Bus Prof Commun Q.* 2012;75(4):453–465. doi:10.1177/1080569912460400
8. Rocco RA, Whalen DJ. Teaching yes, and... improve in sales classes: enhancing student adaptive selling skills, sales performance, and teaching evaluations. *J Mark Educ.* 2014;36(2):197–208. doi:10.1177/0273475314537278
9. Iyengar R. MBA: the soft and hard skills that matter. *IUP Journal of Soft Skills.* 2015;9(1):7–14.
10. Datar SM, Garvin DA, Cullen PG. Rethinking the MBA: business education at a crossroads. *J Manag Dev.* 2011;30(5):451–462. doi:10.1108/02621711111132966
11. Rao T, Saxena S, Chand V, et al. Responding to industry needs: reorienting management education. *Vikalpa,* 2014;39(4):1–10. doi:10.1177/0256090920140401
12. Mintzberg H. *Simply managing: what managers do — and can do better.* San Francisco, CA: Berrett-Koehler Publishers, Inc; 2013.
13. Davidson PL, Calhoun JG, Sinioris ME, Griffith JR. A framework for evaluating and continuously improving the NCHL transformational leadership initiative. *Qual Manag Health Care.* 2002;11(1):3–13. doi:10.1097/00019514-200211010-00005
14. National Center for Healthcare Leadership. *Healthcare leadership competency model 3.0;* Chicago, Illinois; 2018. www.nchl.org/page?page=272
15. Council on Education for Public Health. *Accreditation criteria: Schools of public health & public health programs.* 2016. https://media.ceph.org/wp_assets/2016.Criteria.pdf

PART II

DEFINE

D1. **Situation & Scope**	D2. **Stakeholders, Difficulties, & Problem Areas**	D3. **Issue Statements & Problem Statement**
D1.1 Describe the *situation* D1.2 Scope the work	D2.1 Begin stakeholder analysis D2.2 Identify *difficulties* D2.3 Group difficulties into *problem areas*	D3.1 Create *issue statement* for each problem area D3.2 Create overall *problem statement* and vision for future

STUDY

S1. **Root Causes & Alternative Solutions**	S2. **Decision Criteria, Research, & Findings**	S3. **Conclusions**
S1.1 Generate possible root causes S1.2 Generate potential alternative solutions	S2.1 Develop decision criteria S2.2 Determine additional information needed S2.3 Develop *findings* through research S2.4 Review, reflect, and revise approach	S3.1 Collate, analyze, and judge the alternative solutions S3.2 Synthesize judgments into a set of *conclusions*

ACT

A1. **Recommendations & Milestones**	A2. **Communication Strategy & Consensus Building**	A3. **Implementation & Monitoring**
A1.1 Create integrated set of *recommendations* A1.2 Develop key implementation milestones	A2.1 Revisit stakeholder analysis A2.2 Create communication plan A2.3 Implement communication plan and validate approval/consensus of recommendations	A3.1 Develop detailed implementation plan A3.2 Monitor results against key performance indicators

PRACTICE THE DEFINE PHASE

OVERVIEW OF PART II

Part II of the text provides the "how-to" practice chapters for the Define phase to help you learn each of the steps in this phase. There is one practice chapter per step (Chapters 5, 6, and 7), followed by the answer key for the practice activities in each of the Define phase chapters (Chapter 8).

The structure of each practice chapter is as follows:

- A brief overview of the step and its substeps
- The "how-to" of completing each substep
- Key steps to complete each substep
- Tips for completing each substep successfully
- Tools that support writing up your work in each substep
- Activities for you to practice each substep

As you work your way through the "how-to" practice chapters, it will be very helpful for you to go back to Chapter 2, "The Problem-Solving Method," to read its corresponding detailed information regarding the "what" description for each Define phase substep.

Many of the activities use The Spinal Frontier case in Chapter 1, "The Problem Is Not Always What It Seems," for you to practice the Problem-Solving Method. The Activity Key chapter provide answers or suggested responses based on The Spinal Frontier case.

As you complete each chapter, you will complete a written product for each of the substeps in it. Thus, the practice chapters should be completed in order, because the work you complete in each practice chapter is used in the next one. Writing out your work is important for internalizing the Problem-Solving Method. As you gain experience in using it, you will rarely write out the steps—they will instead be a part of your logical thought process.

Leave yourself time for uninterrupted attention to work through each chapter. The activities will require your thoughtful application.

CHAPTER 5

PRACTICE DEFINE STEP D1: SITUATION AND SCOPE

OVERVIEW OF DEFINE PHASE

Part II of the text covers the Define phase of the Problem-Solving Method, shown in Figure 5.1. The Define phase comprises three major steps, each of which has several substeps:

D1: Situation and Scope (Chapter 5, "Practice Define Step D1: Situation and Scope")

D2: Stakeholders, Difficulties, and Problem Areas (Chapter 6, "Practice Define Step D2: Stakeholders, Difficulties and Problem Areas")

D3: Issue Statements and Problem Statement (Chapter 7, "Practice Define Step D3: Issue Statements and Problem Statement")

By the time you have completed Chapter 7, "Practice Define Step D3: Issue Statements and Problem Statement," you will have developed a written product for each of the seven substeps in the Define phase. Each of the written products builds on the previous ones.

DEFINE STEP D1: SITUATION AND SCOPE

As shown in Figure 5.2, there are two substeps in the Situation and Scope step in the Define phase of the Problem-Solving Method: D1.1, Describe the Situation; and D1.2, Scope the Work.

These two substeps are important because they set the stage for the problem-solving process. Thus, it is important to accurately capture the essence of the facts of what is going on that deserve management attention for resolution, and to articulate the deliverable and time frame for solving the problem.

Re-read the Situation and Scope section of Chapter 2, "The Problem-Solving Method" before completing this section. The Activity Key with answers or examples of written products for each of the activities can be found in Chapter 8, "Define Phase Activity Key."

DEFINE

D1. **Situation & Scope**	D2. **Stakeholders, Difficulties, & Problem Areas**	D3. **Issue statements & Problem Statement**
D1.1 Describe the *situation* D1.2 Scope the work	D2.1 Begin stakeholder analysis D2.2 Identify *difficulties* D2.3 Group difficulties into *problem areas*	D3.1 Create *issue statement* for each problem area D3.2 Create overall *problem statement* and vision for future

FIGURE 5.1 Define phase of the Problem-Solving Method.

PRACTICE D1.1: DESCRIBE THE SITUATION

The situation is a description of the difficulties—facts, empirical data, and key stakeholders' opinions—that indicate there is a difference between "what is" and "what ought to be," along with the context of the situation and the key stakeholders involved.

HOW TO DESCRIBE THE SITUATION

The situation is a succinct description of the problem that captures the difficulties, the context, and the stakeholders. It tells a brief story that describes the problem that is the difference between "what is" and "what ought to be" that needs management attention. It is important that facts be clearly differentiated from opinions in the situation description. This is because, by definition, difficulties must be facts. Thus, any stakeholders' opinions that are included in the situation description must be stated as opinions.

The situation description is created after you conduct preliminary fact finding. You glean information from your initial discussion with the person(s) who has come to you with their concerns. Or you may have identified a problem through reviewing organizational data or reports.

Based on what you learn, you may need to talk to a few other key stakeholders to learn more about their perspectives of the who, what, when, where and why of the problem. This is easier said than done. It takes practice to create a coherent situation description through question asking, observation, and listening skills. This is why people who excel at solving organizational problems often say that being a good problem solver isn't about knowing the right answers, it is about figuring out the right questions to ask of the right people.

DEFINE

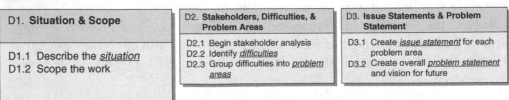

D1. **Situation & Scope**	D2. **Stakeholders, Difficulties, & Problem Areas**	D3. **Issue Statements & Problem Statement**
D1.1 Describe the *situation* D1.2 Scope the work	D2.1 Begin stakeholder analysis D2.2 Identify *difficulties* D2.3 Group difficulties into *problem areas*	D3.1 Create *issue statement* for each problem area D3.2 Create overall *problem statement* and vision for future

FIGURE 5.2 Define step D1: Situation and scope.

The information gathering in this step is at a high-level. It focuses on identifying the difficulties, the context, and the stakeholders. You do not try to identify root causes, you don't analyze potential solutions, and you do not jump to a recommended course of action. The situation description should be no more than a few paragraphs up to a few pages long.

If you are working on a project as a student or a fellow, you should have gathered the information you need to write a situation description within about a week of starting your project. As you gain experience in solving problems, developing an accurate situation description may sometimes take no longer than a few phone calls or a quick meeting to get the information you need, and it will usually not be put in a written format unless the situation is complex.

If you are working on a written case for a course or a case competition, the description from which you will summarize the situation is the case as presented to you.

For your capstone project, summer internship or residency project, or other student consulting projects, you typically will be given a brief written summary of your project prior to your initial meeting with your organizational preceptor, similar to Exhibit 1.1 in Chapter 1, "The Problem Is Not Always What It Seems."

This is usually followed by an initial kickoff meeting with your project preceptor. As part of the meeting discussion, your preceptor will often provide you with names of key stakeholders, or sometimes invite those key stakeholders to the initial meeting.

You need to follow up to interview a few key stakeholders soon after the initial meeting to learn more about the situation. Thus, you are "jumping ahead" to a preliminary start to the stakeholder analysis, substep D2.1 of the Define phase, to help you understand the situation.

Based on the written project summary you received, your kickoff meeting information, and what you learned from early interviews with key stakeholders, you should have the information you need to summarize what you have learned as a situation description.

If you are conducting a project for your fellowship, the beginning of the project may start with a meeting with your mentor or preceptor. Or it may be a situation that arises during a team meeting for which you volunteer to study in more detail.

As you progress in your career, situations that requires problem-solving attention come to light in a variety of ways. It could be a short conversation in the hallway; a check-in meeting with a colleague; a session of rounding or observing; reviewing data, key performance indicators, or reports; a call for consulting services; an assignment to work on a special project; or the emergence of an urgent situation.

In addition to summarizing what your team has learned about the difficulties of the problem to set the stage for the rest of your problem-solving activities, the situation description is often useful when communicating with different stakeholder group audiences in the organization. However, the content and length may need to be revised depending on the audience.

Regarding content, your situation description will, at times, identify the specific stakeholder whose opinion is stated. However, they may have shared things in confidence.

In this case, you should not identify the exact person whose opinion it is, just that it is an opinion that was shared. Additionally, your preceptor may have shared confidential data, strategy decisions, or other information that should not be shared with others. This restriction needs to be honored by your team as you present either internal or external to the organization.

Similarly, the length of the situation description may need to vary depending on the audience with whom it is being shared. For your organizational preceptors, the full situation description is generally needed, with the exception of identifying stakeholders who asked that they not be identified in what they have shared with you.

However, for other stakeholder groups, the full situation description may have too much detail, and should be greatly condensed. This is also true when you present your work in front of an audience. You need to set the stage with an overview of the situation, but not get bogged down in the detail.

KEY STEPS TO DEFINE THE SITUATION

Step 1: When you are conducting a project, come to the kickoff meeting prepared. Read all of the materials provided to you about the project prior to your kickoff meeting. Conduct some preliminary research about the organization and about the general subject of the project as you know it (e.g., joint ventures).

Step 2: After your initial meetings and fact finding, describe the situation by writing down in paragraph form what you have learned are the key difficulties, the context of these difficulties, and the key stakeholders that are affected by the difficulties.

Step 3: Review your written situation description with your faculty advisor (if the project is part of your coursework), and preceptor, mentor, or person in the organization to whom you are reporting for the project, to ensure they are in agreement with it.

TIPS TO DEFINE THE SITUATION

- To better understand the context of the problem, prior to your kickoff meeting, review the website of the organization to understand its history, market share, competitors, financial health, current news or issues, and so forth. You should also read the local newspaper to understand current issues in the organization's local healthcare market.

- Do not get "too deep in the weeds" in your preliminary fact-finding activities to develop your description of the situation. For a capstone or internship/residency project, you should be able to write your initial situation description within a week or so of beginning the project based on your initial fact finding from your project description, your kickoff meeting, your initial interviews with the few key stakeholders, and any organizational reports or data that may have been shared with you.

- The situation should be no longer than a few paragraphs to a few pages long, double spaced.

■ The stakeholder opinions in the situation description you provide to the organization should not identify which specific stakeholder shared this opinion
with you. Keep the sources of the opinions confidential.

TOOL TO DEFINE THE SITUATION

The situation description is at most a few paragraphs long. As such, a tool to support its
development is usually not necessary. You instead work to write a concise summary of
the difficulties of the problem, the stakeholders involved, and the context of the difficulties within the background of the organization at this point in time.

However, when providing updates about your project to various stakeholder groups
in the organization, it can be useful to provide your situation description in the format
of a communication tool that is familiar to them. This helps you translate the Problem-
Solving Method situation description into a structured terminology that is well understood by these key stakeholders.

Ask the organization if they used a structured communication tool. For example, a
communication tool used extensively by clinicians in many healthcare organizations is
the SBAR tool: Situation, Background, Assessment, Recommendations.[1] Pronounced
"S-BAR," the tool, shown in Exhibit 5.1, provides a succinct structured format to facilitate

EXHIBIT 5.1

EXAMPLE SBAR TOOL

S	Situation	
B	Background	
A	Assessment	
R	Recommendation	

the transfer of information. It is frequently used by clinicians to communicate with providers when discussing patients, especially during change of shift.

In the clinical use of SBAR, the Situation is a brief description of the patient's problem—the reason a clinician is communicating with another clinician about a patient's condition. The Background is the context and brief history about the patient's diagnosis and relevant medical history to the current problem. The Assessment is the set of quantitative and qualitative facts about the patient relevant to the current situation, such as vital signs and recent laboratory results, along with a clinical judgment or possible diagnosis of what might be wrong with the patient. The Recommendation is the next step for the patient's care plan—a clear articulation by the speaker of the request for how to move the patient's care forward.[1]

If you elect to use an SBAR format for your project's situation description, you would have only enough information at Step D1.1 to complete the Situation and Background portions. The Situation would briefly describe the difficulties and the stakeholders involved, while the Background would describe why this set of difficulties is arising or relevant to the organization at this point in time.

You would not have the information needed for the Assessment summary until after you complete the Study phase of the Problem-Solving Method, and the Recommendations could not be completed until you have developed your recommendations in the Act phase.

ACTIVITIES TO DEFINE THE SITUATION

Use The Spinal Frontier case in Chapter 1, "The Problem Is Not Always What It Seems," for the Application Activities.

DEFINE ACTIVITY 1

Read through The Spinal Frontier case several times. Then, critique the situation description below.

- Which "facts" are inaccurate as stated and why? How could they be rewritten to make them facts?

- What phrases are opinions that need to be rewritten so that they are stated as facts?

- Which statements should be omitted because they are not difficulties?

- Which statements should be rewritten for the situation description shared with the organization to protect the confidentiality of what was said by key stakeholders that were interviewed?

- Are there any difficulties that have been omitted?

■ THE SPINAL FRONTIER SITUATION DESCRIPTION

Prism Health System, a highly integrated system in the Midwest that also owns its own health plan, is publicly committed to the Triple Aim. The Health System needs to reduce the cost of providing care to patients with chronic musculoskeletal issues. They started a musculoskeletal service line 2 years ago, led by a physician-administrator dyad, to coordinate musculoskeletal care across the continuum. But their costs are still too high. Because the dyad leadership team needs better information to manage the service line, they were surprised when they were told that their costs were too high by the health plan CEO. If Prism Health System can't successfully reduce their costs, the Prism health plan CEO threatened the health system COO that the health system will not be the preferred partner with the health plan on a Spine Center of Distinction Program.

To reduce costs, Prism Health System is planning to enter into a joint venture with MedSpine, a national provider that specializes in low-cost, high quality spine care, as documented in peer-reviewed articles. They have received a joint venture proposal from MedSpine, and the Health System COO said that it looks profitable. However, several key stakeholders are not on board with the joint venture, and the service line leadership has been ignoring their concerns.

The physician-administrator service line dyad leaders are moving too fast, and they aren't engaging in the due diligence required for joint ventures. The hospital CFO is opposed because the joint venture will hurt the hospital financially. The Director of Physical Therapy is opposed because she will have to lay off staff. The Spine Surgeon is not clear why they want to reduce spine surgical volume, since this is what he was hired to do. He is also upset because the joint venture hasn't even been discussed with the service line steering committee.

The service line leadership team and the health system COO need to convince these key stakeholders that a joint venture is the right strategy to pursue to reduce costs. The health system will also need to start rewarding its clinical and administrative leaders for value rather than volume and revenue production to achieve the Triple Aim.

DEFINE ACTIVITY 2

After reviewing your responses and the answers in Chapter 8, "Define Phase Activity Key," for Activity 1, write a situation description that accurately captures the difficulties, the context, and the key stakeholders. Are there both short-term and long-term issues in the situation? What are they? If you had to describe the key issue in the case, what is it?

DEFINE ACTIVITY 3

Briefly summarize your situation description for the Situation and Background sections of an SBAR format. Each should be no longer than a few sentences that would be relevant for a quick overview of the situation and background.

DEFINE ACTIVITY 4

Read the section called *Now What?* in Chapter 1, "The Problem Is Not Always What It Seems." The students were at an impasse when they emailed their faculty advisor. But now that you are practicing the first step of the Problem-Solving Method, role play the meeting with the faculty advisor using the the situation description you developed in Activity 2.

How might the student team clarify the situation with their faculty advisor before approaching the organization again? What should be the students' goal for the meeting with their faculty advisor?

DEFINE ACTIVITY 5

As a student or early graduate, you may have limited real-world knowledge about the topic in your case or project. This can make it difficult to understand the context in which the problem resides. It is helpful to conduct literature and Internet searches and talk with industry contacts and experts to learn more about the topics and terminology in your case or project.

Reading through Exhibit 1.1 in Chapter 1, "The Problem Is Not Always What It Seems," what contextual knowledge would be helpful for you to have researched prior to your kickoff meeting?

PRACTICE D1.2: SCOPE THE WORK

The scope of work is a clear articulation of the deliverable expected of the person or team solving the problem, the due date of the deliverable, and the time (and budget) to be allocated to the problem-solving process.

HOW TO SCOPE THE WORK

If you are using a written case in class or for a case competition, then it, or the case discussion questions, typically includes a description of the scope of work.

In student projects completed in organizations, there is a need for mutual agreement among the student team members, the organizational preceptor or key decision maker, and the faculty advisor on the final product that is expected to be delivered.

It is important that the deliverable is a reasonable expectation given the time frame of the project. For example, if the capstone project is completed over the course of a semester, then the deliverable must be able to be completed in that time frame. If a part of the deliverable requires organizational data that cannot be made available in that time frame, then it will need to be excluded from the scope of work.

A summary statement in a written project description is usually provided to the student team at the start of the project regarding what the organization sees as its expected deliverable. At the kickoff meeting, the deliverable and elements of the scope of work should be discussed. An example consulting agreement in the tools section that follows provides a summary of the types of issues covered in a scope of work document. Within about a week or so of starting your project, you should complete a scope of work document that is signed by all responsible parties. In some projects, there might be an executive sponsor of the project who assumes overall responsibility for it within the organization, but this person will delegate the ongoing interaction with the student team to a project preceptor. In other cases the sponsor and the preceptor will be the same person.

As you work through the steps of the Problem-Solving Method, you will often uncover new difficulties in the situation that were not evident at the outset. If this happens, you need to make the project sponsors in the organization aware of what you have uncovered.

If these new difficulties materially affect the trajectory of the project, the scope may need to be renegotiated. That is, if something new is added to the scope, or the expected deliverable changes based on new information, then the scope may need to be renegotiated. Otherwise, you may find yourself in what project management terminology is called "scope creep." This happens when new things get added to the expected deliverable, but the resources and time frame available do not. Scope creep should be avoided.

In a real-world situation, the scope of work is driven by a variety of factors. Time and organizational resources are usually major factors that determine the breadth and depth of what will be included and excluded from the problem-solving work.

As a leader experienced in solving problems, when you are presented with a set of difficulties, you will automatically begin generating a situation description in your head of what is going on. Then, based on what you are hearing or reading, you will identify what is needed in terms of a deliverable. Is this a crisis situation for which an immediate decision is needed? Is it a complex situation that will require assembling a team to investigate to arrive at a set of recommendations?

As you develop problem-solving expertise, you will be able to sort out and make conscious decisions about what parts of the problem should be addressed now, and what parts to postpone or eliminate entirely.

KEY STEPS TO SCOPE THE WORK

Step 1: Review the initial project description, and your notes from your kickoff meeting, preliminary interviews, and any initial data or reports provided to you by the organization. As you do this review, identify the scope of work elements of your project that you will need to define such as desired deliverable, timeline, budget, team(s) involved, communication cadence, what areas of the organizations or topics are in and out of scope, and so on.

Step 2: Determine what format you will use for a scope of work document. The organization may have a preferred template for you to use. Or use the example consulting agreement document for student projects provided in the tools that follow.

Step 3: Complete a written scope of work by articulating the possible points: organizational sponsors, team, deliverable, timeline, deadlines, meeting cadence, budget. Also articulate any team or organizational resource constraints faced by your team.

Step 5: Discuss the agreement with your project sponsors and your faculty advisor, and revise if needed to seek agreement. Signatures are strongly encouraged as a way to signify that all are in agreement.

TIPS TO SCOPE THE WORK

- One of your team members should be listed as the project manager to facilitate communication between the organization and your team. Communication (email, phone calls) between the organization and the team would be directed to the student identified as the project manager.

- Recognize that there probably will be pieces missing in the agreement at this time that you can agree to circle back to at certain milestones during the project.

- This is your opportunity to brand yourselves as a consulting team from your university. Provide professional looking resumes or biographical sketches to the stakeholders at the kickoff meeting so they know who you are.

- Additionally, think ahead about how you want to brand your presentation. Seek proper permissions through your faculty adviser to include your university logo and branding on any documents and reports shared with the organization. Or the organization may have branded PowerPoint templates that they want you to use as a template.

TOOL TO SCOPE THE WORK

Exhibit 5.2 is an example project consulting agreement template that shows the general areas of documentation included in a scope of work. This can be used in whole or adapted for your needs.

EXHIBIT 5.2

EXAMPLE PROJECT CONSULTING AGREEMENT

PROJECT CONSULTING AGREEMENT

DATE:	[date]
PROJECT:	[title of project]
EXECUTIVE SPONSOR:	[name, title, phone number, and email of executive in organization sponsoring the project]
SITE PRECEPTOR:	[may be same person as sponsor, but if there are additional organization preceptors, list here]
PROJECT TEAM:	[names and contact information for each student team member, indicate which team member is the project manager]
PROJECT BACKGROUND:	[brief description of existing condition of project – three or four sentences]

(continued)

EXHIBIT 5.2

EXAMPLE PROJECT CONSULTING AGREEMENT (*CONTINUED*)

PROJECT DELIVERABLE:	[indicate core purpose and deliverable of project in one or two sentences; answer the question, "What are you doing for your project?"
PROJECT SCOPE:	[indicate areas/departments/processes included in the project and areas that are explicitly not included]
PROBLEM STATEMENT:	[initial construct of problem statement for project]
CONSTRAINTS:	[standard constraints (limited time, availability of data, etc.) and also list any foreseeable barriers to completing the project]
APPROACH:	[indicate basic tools or techniques you will use to address problem (quantitative and qualitative) and how the data will be obtained; list overview of initial research plan with milestones (interviews and data); list any confidentiality agreements needed and when they will be completed]
ROLE OF PROJECT TEAM:	[create list of team responsibilities – i.e., manage the project timeline and produce deliverables, perform analyses described previously and summarize results, provide periodic updates to project sponsor(s) as necessary, etc.]
ROLE OF SPONSOR(S):	[create list of sponsor responsibilities; i.e., establish and communicate the guidelines and objectives of the project, facilitate data access, participate in goal setting with the project team, monitor the progress of the project, etc.]
ESTIMATED START DATE:	[date]
FINAL SITE PRESENTATION:	[time, and location that final deliverable will be presented]
SCHEDULE OF DELIVERABLES:	[list approximate schedule of deliverables in chronological order; include all final deliverables (written reports, presentations, etc.) and interim update reports]
CRITERIA FOR SUCCESS:	[identify two to four factors that will determine whether project is successful]
FOLLOW-UP:	[suggested language: "The project team will not be available for additional work or implementation; however, the final product will provide appropriate implementation plans and/or guidelines for further study of the problem."]

AGREED (Signatures):

_____   _____
SITE PRECEPTOR   Date   STUDENT PROJECT MANAGER   Date

_____   _____
EXECUTIVE SPONSOR   Date   FACULTY ADVISOR   Date

ACTIVITIES TO SCOPE THE WORK

Use The Spinal Frontier case in Chapter 1, "The Problem Is Not Always What It Seems," for the Application Activities.

DEFINE ACTIVITY 6

Given the situation description you developed in Activity 2 (or provided in the Chapter 8, "Define Phase Activity Key" for Activity 2), how should the following project deliverable summary be revised for discussion with the project preceptors at Prism Health System?

■ SCOPE OF WORK SUMMARY IN NEED OF REVISION

Our project team will develop an implementation plan for the joint venture with Med-Spine in a way that convinces the key stakeholders (the dyad leaders, the system COO, the hospital CFO, the Director of Physical Therapy, the CEO of the health plan, the Spine Surgeon, and patients and the community) that a joint venture is the best solution moving forward.

DEFINE ACTIVITY 7

Role play a follow-up meeting with the Prism organization to discuss what you have learned so far and the implications for the scope of work for your project. What is your goal for that meeting?

DEFINE ACTIVITY 8

Assume that Prism Health System and your student consulting team came to an agreement on your situation description and revised the deliverable in Activity 6 scope of work that you provided to them.

Using either the example Project Consulting Agreement provided in Exhibit 5.2, or another project scope document of your choice, complete the consulting agreement as if you are the student team.

REFERENCE

1. Institute for Healthcare Improvement. *SBAR: Situation-background-assessment-recommendation*. (2017) http://lsqin.org/wp-content/uploads/2017/08/SBARTechniqueforCommunication.pdf

CHAPTER 6

PRACTICE DEFINE STEP D2: STAKEHOLDERS, DIFFICULTIES, AND PROBLEM AREAS

DEFINE STEP D2: STAKEHOLDERS, DIFFICULTIES, AND PROBLEM AREAS

As shown in Figure 6.1, there are three substeps in the Stakeholders, Difficulties, and Problem Areas step in the Define phase of the Problem-Solving Method: D2.1, Begin stakeholder analysis; D2.2, Identify difficulties; and D2.3, Group difficulties into problem areas.

These three substeps are critical for your problem-solving efforts, as they are the ones that help you "make the problem bigger" to ensure that you have captured all of the interrelated aspects of the problem that need management attention for resolution.

As you develop your expertise in solving problems, you learn how to elicit and identify difficulties by asking the right questions of the right stakeholders to mentally complete a stakeholder analysis, and determine what readily available data to review. As you listen and observe, it becomes second nature in your thought process to be able to quickly sort out which difficulties are facts and which are opinions.

Then, in the problem areas substep of Define phase step D2, you begin to engage in convergent thinking by reviewing the difficulties you identified and to group them based on their similarity into buckets called problem areas. This helps you condense the difficulties into a handful of areas on which you can focus your efforts in the remainder of the Problem-Solving Method.

Reread the Define Step D2 section in Chapter 2 before completing this section. The Activity Key with answers or examples of written products for each of the activities can be found in Chapter 8.

PRACTICE D2.1: BEGIN STAKEHOLDER ANALYSIS

The stakeholder analysis identifies all the persons and groups affected by the situation and frames the problem from their various points of view.

DEFINE

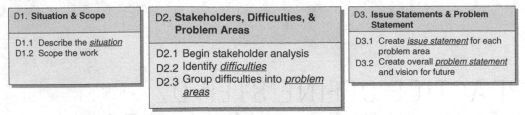

FIGURE 6.1 Define step D2: Stakeholders, difficulties, and problem areas.

HOW TO BEGIN THE STAKEHOLDER ANALYSIS

You may have already had some initial conversations with a limited number of key stakeholders prior to this step as you developed an understanding of the situation and determined the scope of work in Define step D1. But it is in this step that you focus on gaining a more complete understanding of the problem from the key stakeholders' points of view.

This provides you with insights into their perceptions of the problem and its history, how it is affecting their work, the difficulties, the perceived root causes, their preferred solutions, and their goals for seeing the problem resolved. In engaging with your key stakeholders, you might uncover additional major difficulties that could require circling back to expand upon or change the description and scope of work in Define step D1. If this occurs, it should be discussed with your preceptor or boss to revise the scope if necessary.

For student projects, the organizational preceptor will usually have let relevant stakeholders in the organization know that they are hosting a student consulting project, and will provide you with organizational stakeholder names and contact information. When you contact the stakeholders to arrange a time to meet with them, include a brief introduction of who you are, and provide a brief explanation of your work.

This is where the brief Situation and Background of an SBAR described in the Define step D1.1 activity can be helpful. You should also include a list of the questions you will be talking about with them and, broadly speaking, what you will be doing with the information they share with you.

The organizational preceptor should review your questions prior to your sending them out. They may have some additional background information that will be helpful to you, and they may suggest some questions that you had not thought about.

When you meet with the stakeholders, they may, in turn, recommend that you speak to others in the organization who have relevant information for you but who are not on your contact list. You want to create a list of these stakeholders, and clarify with your preceptors whether these additional stakeholders know of your project, and whether you have permission to contact them.

The stakeholders may also mention organizational data or reports, or external experts that will be of use to you during your Study phase of the Problem-Solving Method. If so, make a note to yourself to follow up with your organizational preceptor about gaining access or contact information for these resources.

For each stakeholder, you develop a list of questions you will be asking that will serve as your interview guide for the conversation. Example questions are in Exhibit 6.1.

Remember that during your interviews, you need to engage in divergent thinking by not contradicting what you are hearing from the stakeholders. You should ask clarifying questions to understand their perspective, but you should be respectful and listen to what they are telling you. Do not argue about the facts during the interview. During the Study phase of the Problem-Solving Method, you will be able to sort out if their opinion is based in fact.

You should take notes during each conversation. These notes are for your use, and are not shared with the organization. While the interview is fresh in your mind, review your notes and expand upon and clarify them as needed.

Then, for each stakeholder, complete one row of the stakeholder analysis table (see Table 6.1 below) to summarize your conversation. Your stakeholder analysis table should have as many completed rows as there are stakeholders interviewed. This tool is used for your own summary, and not shared with the organization.

You will use the stakeholder analysis table as an analysis tool that you circle back to as you work through the steps of the Problem-Solving Method. There are a number of ways you will use the stakeholder analysis.

First, it summarizes in one location what you have learned from all of your stakeholders. Review it for accuracy and completeness.

Second, it helps you identify and understand the difficulties in the situation that describe the "mess" that is the problem.

Third, you need to study and analyze the stakeholder analysis table to make sure you understand the similarities and differences between the stakeholders' perceptions and opinions to see where there are conflicting points of view. You need to pay particular attention to where there are differences in perceptions and opinions to understand what is driving them. Is it a difference in goals? In values? In facts used? These differences highlight where you will especially want to gather additional data to clarify facts in the Study phase of the Problem-Solving Method.

Fourth, it provides you with starting lists of possible root causes of the difficulties and potential alternative solutions in the first step of the Study phase.

Fifth, as you complete the Study phase, the stakeholder analysis table will continue to be expanded, changed, and revised as needed.

Finally, it gets you to start thinking about the communications plan you will need in order to gain approval of your recommendations in the Act phase of the Problem-Solving Method.

As you gain experience in solving problems in real-world organizations, you will learn how to identify the key stakeholders with whom you need to engage for your stakeholder analysis. You will rarely complete a written stakeholder analysis table. However, the column headings of the stakeholder analysis table provide the framework of the information you are seeking as you talk with stakeholders. Again, you will especially listen for where there are differences in perceptions and opinions to clue you in about where you need to focus particular attention during the Study phase to sort out the facts.

If you are working with a paper case for a class, the stakeholders are identified in the case. Because the cases are fictitious, you may be wondering how you can interview the stakeholders. The obvious answer is you can't. So, when working with a fictitious case, you are allowed to "assume" what the stakeholders would say in two different ways.

First, read the information provided about the various stakeholders in the case, and then complete the cells of the stakeholder analysis table where you can. Second, contact your mentor to ask them how a stakeholder in a given role might respond. Or your mentor may be able to connect you with someone in their organization with a similar role so that you can ask them. This will enable you to complete the stakeholder analysis table.

KEY STEPS TO BEGIN THE STAKEHOLDER ANALYSIS

Step 1: Review the situation description and scope of work to identify and list out the stakeholders, including both individual stakeholders and groups of stakeholders. Remember that the key stakeholders include:

- Those who are affected by the problem
- Those who will be approving your final recommendations either through formal vote or informal consensus
- Those who will be responsible for implementing the solutions to fix the problem
- Those who may be affected by the changes resulting from solutions implemented to fix the problem
- Patients and their families, and the community served by the organization, are always stakeholders
- The CEO of the organization and the Board of Directors are always stakeholders, as "the buck stops with them"

Step 2: Create interview guides for each major stakeholder group. An example interview guide is provided in Exhibit 6.1, although the subset of questions you would ask from the example interview guide would vary by stakeholder group.

Step 3: Share the stakeholder list and your interview guides with the organizational preceptor and develop a plan to schedule meetings with stakeholders, observe processes, and receive preliminary organizational data.

Step 4: Begin to interview stakeholders, observe processes, if relevant, and review preliminary data.

Step 5: Summarize the information you gather from your stakeholders into a stakeholder analysis table. You update the table as you continue to learn from your stakeholders as you work through the steps of the Problem-Solving Method.

TIPS TO BEGIN THE STAKEHOLDER ANALYSIS

- Be as specific as possible when listing stakeholders. For instance, if different physician specialty groups view the problem differently (e.g., Emergency Department physicians versus Admitting physicians), they should be listed as separate stakeholders in the stakeholder analysis table.

- In healthcare situations, patients, their families, and the community served by the healthcare organization should always be listed as stakeholders. If you do not have the opportunity to talk with them directly, you should ask other stakeholders who interact with them. And, remember we are all patients and we are all family members. Interview each other, ask your colleagues or mentor, and ask your family members. To better understand the community served, read the local newspaper.

- Share your interview guides with your preceptors prior to your interviews for feedback. Also share a list of any additional stakeholders for potential interviews not identified on the initial list agreed upon. This is to ensure there are no surprises on the part of the organizational preceptor.

- Email your interview guide to the stakeholder prior to your meeting to give them enough time to review and think about the questions. This can lead to better conversations, and the stakeholder will often invite others to the meeting who could provide helpful insights or data based on the interview guide questions.

- Meet face-to-face for your stakeholder interviews as much as possible. Do not rely on email or computer interviews as a way to interview stakeholders. Make a human connection.

- Be sure to introduce yourselves and your purpose prior to asking your questions. Describe how their answers will not be attributed to them to maintain their confidentiality. Your team will want honest feedback, and it is okay to let your interviewees know you will not be sharing their feedback in a way that would identify them without their permission.

- It is helpful to have two team members participate when conducting the stakeholder interviews. One asks the questions, the other writes the answers. The one writing the answers also keeps track to make sure all questions in the interview guide are getting asked, and serves as the timekeeper to keep the conversation on track to get the interview completed in the time available. This is important because the person being interviewed can sometimes start veering into areas that aren't directly relevant to the situation you have been asked to address, and you need to gently steer the conversation back to the topic at hand.

- When asking stakeholders about possible root causes or potential alternative solutions, it can sometimes put them on the defensive if you ask them "why" they think something. It can help to instead ask "help me understand" or "what reasons might there be" or "do you have an example or could I observe the process or data to help me better understand" for something they stated.

■ Your specific interview notes and your stakeholder analysis table are not provided to your organizational preceptor. What is shared with the organization is a summary of the stakeholder analysis that de-identifies what any specific stakeholder has shared with you.

TOOL TO BEGIN THE STAKEHOLDER ANALYSIS

An example interview guide of sample questions for the stakeholders in The Spinal Frontier case in Chapter 1 is in Exhibit 6.1. You do not ask all the questions of all stakeholders. For example, questions for front line staff may relate more to patient care, barriers to providing the best care, and opportunity to observe work and patient flow. Leadership questions would likely be more about the mission, the scope of services, strategic direction, provider relations, future ideas, and so forth.

EXHIBIT 6.1

SAMPLE INTERVIEW GUIDE FOR THE SPINAL FRONTIER CASE

INTERVIEWEE INFORMATION

Name	
Area/Group	
Role/Responsibilities	
Interview Date	

INTRODUCTION
We are a student team working with your organization this semester to arrive at a set of recommendations for how it might best position itself to be the provider of choice in the community for musculoskeletal care. As part of our work, we are seeking information on your perceptions of the Prism Health System's Musculoskeletal Clinical Service Line and how it might best be positioned to ensure it remains competitive in today's value based healthcare market.

INTERVIEW OBJECTIVES
We have prepared a set of questions to help guide the discussion. The objective of these questions is to gain your insight regarding:

• Organizational and market information related to the Musculoskeletal Clinical Service Line
• Current efficiency/effectiveness of the Musculoskeletal Clinical Service Line and future opportunities
• Musculoskeletal Clinical Service Line revenue and growth opportunities

The insights gained during our interviews with key stakeholders will be synthesized and summarized to establish qualitative and quantitative conclusions and recommendations regarding the future direction of the Service Line.

(continued)

EXHIBIT 6.1

SAMPLE INTERVIEW GUIDE FOR THE SPINAL FRONTIER CASE (*CONTINUED*)

INTERVIEW QUESTIONS
(Note, MCSL = Musculoskeletal Clinical Service Line)

Prism Health System and MCSL: Please describe:

1. Your role at Prism Health System and the MCSL.
2. Prism's mission, vision, values, and strategy and how your role supports them.
3. Prism's market-competition, payer landscape, government involvement, technology forces, community profile.
4. Services provided by the MCSL to the community and the community perceptions of them.
5. How Prism's services for chronic musculoskeletal issues compare to competitors in the community, and the key differentiators of Prism's MCSL care.
6. The components across the continuum of care in the MCSL and the patient journey, any opportunities in improving the continuity of care, any changes on the horizon, and rationale for these changes.
7. The patients being treated by the MCSL and any improvement initiatives/innovations that are underway or that you would suggest (in terms of patients by diagnosis in different services). Rationale for suggested improvements/innovations.
8. The intended outcomes for the MCSL and for its patients. Are those outcomes being achieved? If not, possible reasons?
9. Quality improvement initiatives underway to drive improvements in quality and costs of care for patients with chronic musculoskeletal issues.
10. The coordination of MCSL care between providers and departments, and how patients move through the MCSL continuum. What is working and what isn't in the coordination of care across the continuum?
11. What does success look like for the MCSL, both now and into the future. Are the metrics of success currently being achieved? If yes, what has facilitated success. If no, what are the barriers?
12. The size of growth opportunity for musculoskeletal services in terms of volume, revenue, products, or services provided.
13. The strengths, weaknesses, opportunities, and threats to the MCSL.
14. The external forces in the market impacting the MCSL.
15. Pros and cons of a joint venture with MedSpine and why, especially in the context of the answers to questions 13 and 14 above.
16. MCSL leadership (clinical and administrative) and how they intersect with payers or other referring physician groups or other affiliations.
17. Who are the providers referring to and participating in the MCSL episode of care.
18. How negotiation with payers specifically will need to be or already are aligned with value-based care.
19. What a shared savings program could look like for the MCSL.

Payer Relations: Please describe:
20. The payer landscape, Prism's payer relations strategy and infrastructure.

SAMPLE INTERVIEW GUIDE FOR THE SPINAL FRONTIER CASE (*CONTINUED*)

21. The employers in the market and Prism's employer relations strategy and infrastructure.
22. The typical insurance package and patient responsibility for payment in terms of copays and deductibles.
23. Existing terms of the major payers' contracts.
24. What has worked and not worked during previous payer negotiations.
25. The existing financial performance of Prism's health plan and their reimbursement, and how this compares to other payers.
26. How pre-authorizations, denials, and/or underpayments are managed with payers.
27. The cost drivers that the health plan asks you about, especially related to the MCSL.

General Summary:

28. Ask for organizational charts of the Prism Health System, the Prism Health Plan, the service lines, and the hospital.
29. Any organizational, cultural, or workflow challenges or barriers to success related to the future of the MCSL.
30. Anything we didn't ask or talk about with you regarding the MCSL that you think we should know.
31. Do you have any questions for us?

After you complete each interview, review your notes for accuracy and completeness, and revise them as necessary. Next, complete a row in the stakeholder analysis table as shown in Table 6.1. Each stakeholder you interview will have their information summarized in a row of the table. For each stakeholder, summarize their goal for the situation being successfully resolved, their perceived difficulties about what is going on in the problem, their perceptions about the root causes of the difficulties, and their preferred solutions to alleviate the problem that would help them achieve their goal.

The last column of the table, called Additional Insights Provided, is where you include any tips or additional insights they may have shared. For example, they may recommend you talk to other stakeholders in the organization that they name, they may tell you about an organizational report that has information relevant to the problem, or they may recommend a contact or expert in the field who would be helpful for you to interview. Recording this information in the table helps you summarize resources for the Study phase, and reminds you of who gave you that insight in case you want to circle back with them.

ACTIVITIES TO BEGIN THE STAKEHOLDER ANALYSIS

Use The Spinal Frontier case in Chapter 1 for the Application Activities.

TABLE 6.1 Stakeholder Analysis Table

STAKEHOLDER	GOAL	PERCEIVED DIFFICULTIES	PERCEIVED ROOT CAUSES (WHY?)	SUGGESTED ALTERNATIVE SOLUTIONS	ADDITIONAL INSIGHTS PROVIDED

■ DEFINE ACTIVITY 9

Create a list of all of the stakeholders and their roles in The Spinal Frontier case. Be sure to identify which stakeholders are members of the Service Line Steering Committee as one of their roles. Remember that there may be stakeholders in the situation who are not specifically named in the case; for example, Prism Health System's CEO and Board of Directors, patients and their families, and the community.

■ DEFINE ACTIVITY 10

Complete a stakeholder analysis table to the best of your ability given the information presented in The Spinal Frontier case.

■ DEFINE ACTIVITY 11

Which of the questions in the interview guide in Exhibit 6.1 would you ask of the Dyad Leadership Team of the Musculoskeletal Clinical Service Line? Which of the questions would you ask of the Director of Physical Therapy? Are there any questions that you think are missing from the interview guide that should be asked of either of these stakeholders?

■ DEFINE ACTIVITY 12

Practice interviewing an administrative or clinical leader, or front line staff in a local healthcare organization using your questions. Ask them to role play answers as if they are a particular stakeholder in the case.

Take notes during the interview. Soon after completing the interview, review, revise, and summarize your notes. Then, complete a row of the stakeholder analysis table.

If multiple students interview different people, summarize the interviews into one stakeholder analysis table.

Discuss the similarities and differences in the perceptions and opinions across the stakeholders.

What are the implications for these differences when you complete the Study and Act phases of the Problem-Solving Method?

PRACTICE D2.2: IDENTIFY DIFFICULTIES

A difficulty is a fact or an opinion that identifies or implies a gap, or difference, between what the situation is, and what it ought to be. In order for an opinion to be a fact, it has to be stated in the difficulty whose opinion it is.

HOW TO IDENTIFY DIFFICULTIES

For your project, there are a variety of sources that you use to identify the difficulties. These include the initial project description you receive prior to your kickoff meeting, the situation description you create, your stakeholder interview notes and analysis table, and any preliminary data shared with you by the organization.

As you review your notes and other sources, write down each difficulty separately, either as a numbered list, or on sticky notes. If the difficulty is an opinion, remember to state whose opinion it is, so that facts can be clearly differentiated from opinions. And, remember, do not speculate about root causes or alternative solutions at this step. Just stick to the facts as presented. Never assume.

When you are done with this step, you will have created a list of all of the difficulties in the situation. It is important to capture all of the difficulties, because otherwise you risk missing an important problem area, which you will develop next in Define substep D2.3.

With experience, you will mentally collate facts and opinions in your head in real time, and automatically sort out which are facts versus opinions. You will be able to listen carefully when a stakeholder comes to you with a concern or complaint, you will regularly make rounds to talk to your employees and observe processes, and you will review organizational data as part of your responsibilities that trigger to you that there are difficulties that may need attention or correction. Is the situation as it should be? Is there a difference between "what is" and "what ought to be?" You will rarely write down the difficulties or fill out a stakeholder analysis table, but you will still complete them in your head.

If you are working with a paper case for a class, you identify the difficulties by reading for sentences or phrases in the case that indicate that there is a difference between "what is" and "what ought to be." It is helpful to read through the case several times. The first time through, just read the case. Then, read the case again, but this time, use a highlighter to identify the difficulties. Then read the case one more time to make sure you identified all of the difficulties. Once you have done this, you can create either a numbered list of difficulties, or write them on sticky notes, one difficulty per sticky note.

You now have a list of the difficulties.

KEY STEPS TO IDENTIFY DIFFICULTIES

Step 1: During your initial and future stakeholder interviews as well as any document or data reviews, listen and probe to identify specific difficulties.

Step 2: With your team, identify and write out the difficulties onto sticky notes and/or put them all in a numbered list in one document. Be sure that difficulties that are opinions indicate whose opinion it is when writing out that difficulty.

TIPS TO IDENTIFY DIFFICULTIES

- Listening carefully at organizational meetings and directly observing processes can be as helpful in identifying difficulties as interviewing stakeholders and reviewing preliminary organizational data. Reading meeting minutes of any committees relevant to the situation is also helpful. Always try to use multiple methods to identify difficulties as time allows.

- As you read through your stakeholder interview notes, review organizational data, and observe processes and meetings, you may uncover difficulties that are tangential to the situation you have been asked by the organization to resolve. Use your scope of work document to help you avoid scope creep. You need to focus on the difficulties that could affect the successful resolution of the problem at hand.

- Team meetings for your student project are more productive if you do preparatory prework prior to your meetings. To develop your skills in identifying difficulties, you should each generate your list of difficulties on your own prior to the team meeting, and come prepared with your list.

TOOL TO IDENTIFY DIFFICULTIES

Because the difficulties will be grouped based on similarity to develop problem areas in substep D2.3 of the Define phase, it is helpful to use sticky notes as a tool to facilitate that process. Write one difficulty per sticky note, and place them on a wall or white board in any order. Figure 6.2 shows some of the difficulties from The Spinal Frontier case listed on sticky notes as an example.

ACTIVITIES TO IDENTIFY DIFFICULTIES

Use The Spinal Frontier case in Chapter 1 for the Application Activities.

■ DEFINE ACTIVITY 13

Using the definition of a difficulty, which of the following statements below are *not* difficulties? Provide a justification for your answers.

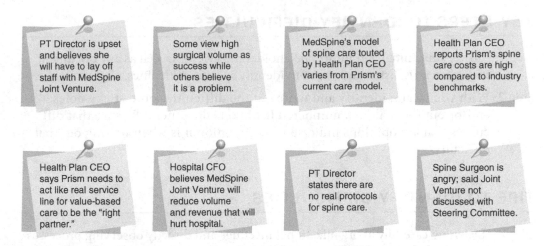

FIGURE 6.2 Sticky notes listing difficulties in The Spinal Frontier case.

1. Prism Health System needs to reduce the cost of providing care to patients with chronic musculoskeletal care needs.

2. Health Plan CEO indicates Prism costs for patients with chronic musculoskeletal care needs are high compared to insurance industry benchmarks.

3. The MedSpine proposal will financially harm the hospital because it will result in layoffs and decreased revenues.

4. The Administrative Dyad Partner of the Musculoskeletal Clinical Service Line was surprised when told by the Health Plan CEO that their costs of care were higher than industry benchmarks.

5. The Health Plan CEO is overstepping his bounds when telling the Health System to talk with MedSpine.

6. The organization needs to look at all their data before deciding what to do.

7. Some stakeholders view increasing utilization for musculoskeletal services as a success, while others perceive that as a problem given Prism's commitment to the Triple Aim.

8. The hospital does not have protocols for managing patients with musculoskeletal issues.

9. The Hospital CFO believes that the MedSpine proposal will hurt the hospital financially.

10. The Physical Therapy Department should be part of the Musculoskeletal Clinical Service Line to improve continuity of care.

11. Many stakeholders feel that the administrator of the Musculoskeletal Clinical Service Line is not listening to them.

12. This major strategic MedSpine joint venture decision was made outside of the committee structure that is intended to provide input into the Musculoskeletal Clinical Service Line.

13. The organization needs better spreadsheets and data to track their costs of care.

14. The Musculoskeletal Clinical Service Line administrator did not know Prism treatment costs were higher than industry standards until told by Health Plan CEO.

15. The Health Plan CEO is telling Prism Health System how to provide clinical care.

16. Prism Health System is not acting like a value-based health system and will be unsuccessful in achieving the Triple Aim.

17. Musculoskeletal Clinical Service Line dyad leaders are not listening to their clinical and financial stakeholders.

18. The stakeholders opposed to the MedSpine proposal don't understand the importance of value-based care to succeed in today's marketplace.

19. Prism Health System should partner with MedSpine to remain competitive in the marketplace.

20. Prism Health system should not partner with MedSpine because of the opposition to the strategic partnership proposal.

■ DEFINE ACTIVITY 14

List all of the difficulties in The Spinal Frontier case. Create a numbered list, or write the difficulties on sticky notes, one per note.

PRACTICE D2.3: GROUP DIFFICULTIES INTO PROBLEM AREAS

Problem areas are sets of key difficulties—facts, empirical data, and stated opinions of key stakeholders—that are grouped based on similarity of evidence that indicate there is a difference between "what is" and "what ought to be."

HOW TO GROUP DIFFICULTIES INTO PROBLEM AREAS

In this substep, you begin to engage in convergent thinking by sorting the difficulties into buckets. To do this, review your list of difficulties and group them into separate buckets based on their similarity or relatedness to each other. These buckets of interrelated difficulties are the problem areas. Although a difficulty can be placed in more than one problem area, try to create buckets of difficulties that are as independent from each other as possible. There are no right or wrong ways to group the difficulties.

If you have created a numbered list of difficulties, you can write down the numbers of the difficulties into separate buckets to group them (e.g., difficulties numbered 1, 5, 7 and 9 are in one bucket). If you have written the difficulties on sticky notes, you can simply take each sticky note, and place it beside the ones that are most similar to it, until you end up with a handful of buckets. If you want to place a difficulty in more than one bucket, then simply write the difficulty again on another sticky note.

Once all of the difficulties have been placed into buckets, read the set of difficulties in each bucket and, based on that set, assign a name to the problem area. If you are having trouble figuring out what to name a problem area, it may suggest that the difficulties in that bucket don't have a common theme to them, and you may need to re-think the difficulties you have included in that bucket. By the end of this substep, each difficulty should have been placed in at least one problem area, and each problem area should have a name.

As you develop experience in using the Problem-Solving Method, you will be able to logically group difficulties mentally into problem areas without the aid of lists or sticky notes. For example, you will be able to listen to a conversation or disagreement during a meeting, discern the difficulties, and then synthesize the difficulties into problem areas as you listen. You can then support moving the group forward either by articulating what you think are the problem areas, or by actually taking them through a facilitated process of listing the difficulties and grouping them into problem areas as part of the group discussion.

KEY STEPS TO GROUP DIFFICULTIES INTO PROBLEM AREAS

Step 1: Group the difficulties into problem areas based on similarity to each other, using either sticky notes or a numbered list of difficulties. Do not name the problem areas until after all the difficulties have been put into a problem area.

Step 2: Review the set of difficulties within each problem area to determine a name for each problem area that succinctly captures the key issue in each problem area; for example, leadership, process, communication, and so on. Generally, you should end up with no more than a handful of problem areas.

Step 3: Go back and review your situation description, your stakeholder analysis, and any other information you have collected through data or observation to ensure you have fully captured all the difficulties and problem areas relevant to the problem you are solving.

TIPS TO GROUP DIFFICULTIES INTO PROBLEM AREAS

- Difficulties can be placed in more than one problem area. However, if there is a great amount of overlap in difficulties between your problem areas, go back and see if you can re-group the difficulties such that the problem areas are as mutually exclusive of each other as possible.

- Do not name the problem areas until after you have grouped the difficulties.

- As you conduct research in the Study phase of the Problem-Solving Method, you may uncover additional difficulties. If these difficulties fit into one of your

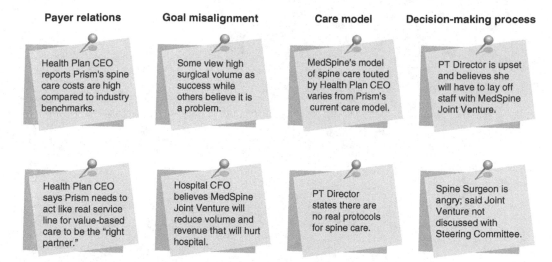

Payer relations	Goal misalignment	Care model	Decision-making process
Health Plan CEO reports Prism's spine care costs are high compared to industry benchmarks.	Some view high surgical volume as success while others believe it is a problem.	MedSpine's model of spine care touted by Health Plan CEO varies from Prism's current care model.	PT Director is upset and believes she will have to lay off staff with MedSpine Joint Venture.
Health Plan CEO says Prism needs to act like real service line for value-based care to be the "right partner."	Hospital CFO believes MedSpine Joint Venture will reduce volume and revenue that will hurt hospital.	PT Director states there are no real protocols for spine care.	Spine Surgeon is angry; said Joint Venture not discussed with Steering Committee.

FIGURE 6.3 Example of problem areas.

problem areas, you should add them. If any of them do not fit, you need to determine if there is a new problem area that affects being able to successfully solve the problem. If there is, the situation description and scope may need to be revised.

TOOL TO GROUP DIFFICULTIES INTO PROBLEM AREAS

If your difficulties are written on sticky notes, group the sticky notes into problem areas on a white board based on their similarity to each other. Review the sticky notes in each problem area to label it with a name that succinctly captures the key issue in the difficulties of that problem area.

If your difficulties are a numbered list, write the numbered list on the white board, and then use the number attached to each difficulty when grouping them. An example of problem areas for The Spinal Frontier case using sticky notes with two difficulties listed for each is shown in Figure 6.3.

ACTIVITIES TO GROUP DIFFICULTIES INTO PROBLEM AREAS

■ DEFINE ACTIVITY 15

You identified the difficulties for The Spinal Frontier case in Activity 14. Group the difficulties you identified into problem areas, and label each problem area with a name.

CHAPTER 7

PRACTICE DEFINE STEP D3: ISSUE STATEMENTS AND PROBLEM STATEMENT

DEFINE STEP D3: ISSUE STATEMENTS AND PROBLEM STATEMENT

As shown in Figure 7.1, there are two substeps in the Issue Statements and Problem Statement step in the Define phase of the Problem-Solving Method: D3.1, Create issue statement for each problem area; and D3.2, Create overall problem statement and vision for the future.

These two substeps are key in the Problem-Solving Method, because it is here that you must accurately define the problem. You do this by accurately identifying the key issue in each problem area, and then summarizing them into a summary statement of the problem and what the organization's future will look like if the problem is successfully resolved.

Reread the Define Step D3 section in Chapter 2 before completing this section. The Activity Key with answers or examples of written products for each of the activities can be found in Chapter 8.

PRACTICE D3.1: CREATE AN ISSUE STATEMENT FOR EACH PROBLEM AREA

An issue statement is the key question that needs to be answered to eliminate, correct, or resolve the set of difficulties in its problem area. An issue statement is required for each problem area. It leads to exploration of action-oriented alternative solutions to resolve that problem area's set of difficulties.

HOW TO CREATE AN ISSUE STATEMENT FOR EACH PROBLEM AREA

In this step, review the set of difficulties in each problem area to identify the key issue that needs resolution. Thus, each problem area requires its own issue statement. The key issue is stated in the form of a question that, if answered, would eliminate or reduce the impact of the difficulties in the problem area.

DEFINE

D1. Situation & Scope	D2. Stakeholders, Difficulties, & Problem Areas	D3. Issue Statements & Problem Statement
D1.1 Describe the *situation* D1.2 Scope the work	D2.1 Begin stakeholder analysis D2.2 Identify *difficulties* D2.3 Group difficulties into *problem areas*	D3.1 Create *issue statement* for each problem area D3.2 Create overall *problem statement* and vision for future

FIGURE 7.1 Define step D3: Issue statements and problem statement.

The question needs to be goal oriented, and it should articulate the barriers to achieving that goal and/or the context in which that goal needs to be achieved. It is not a question of fact or a yes/no question, and it should never have a solution embedded in it. As described in detail in Chapter 2, issue statements are generally structured in one of the two formats that follow.

> *How can (or how should) organization X achieve {stated goal relevant to the set of difficulties in this problem area} in light of {stated barriers that are hindering that goal from being achieved that relate to the vision of the future} and/or {broader organizational goals}?*
>
> *What is the appropriate {structure, goal, or benchmark} for the organization regarding {problem area focus}, and how can the organization best achieve that {structure, goal, or benchmark} in light of {stated barriers} and/or {broader organizational goals}?*

Creating an issue statement that accurately captures the key issue is harder than it seems. A well-articulated issue statement promotes agreement among stakeholders that this is the key question that needs to be answered for that problem area. As you gain experience in teasing out the key issue to resolve in a problem area, you will gain the trust of your colleagues and become recognized as an opinion leader in the organization.

Crafting crisp, clear, cogent issue statements takes practice. Well written issue statements should capture the elements of the situation description such that someone not familiar with it could read your issue statements and be very clear about what is going on. Thus, the issue statements need to articulate the key issues, as well as identify the barriers and context.

For your student project, each team member should independently craft their own issue statement for each problem area. Use either of the formats previously described to write your issue statements. Sometimes, stating the issue statement as a "how" question seems a best fit. At other times, a "what" question may be more logical. Again, it just takes practice.

Once each team member has written their issue statements, you should come together as a group to share and discuss them. Draw upon the best aspects of each of them to arrive at your final set of issue statements, and share them with your organizational preceptor for feedback.

As you gain experience in solving problems, you will develop the ability to quickly synthesize the key issues after mentally identifying difficulties and grouping them into problem areas in real time. If you are working with a team that is struggling to identify the problem that needs to be solved, facilitating them through a team exercise of identifying difficulties, grouping them into problem areas, naming the problem areas, and writing issue statements, can result in moving the team's problem-solving progress forward. This helps the team from prematurely jumping to solutions. The goal at this step is to ask the right questions to identify the problem to be solved, not argue about whose preferred solution is best.

After writing the issue statements, review your problem areas to see if they have a logical priority to them, or a logical cascade, in that the best acceptable alternative to one problem area will drive the best acceptable alternative in another problem area. If one does seem to be the first order problem area, make sure it is the first problem area listed in your problem list.

KEY STEPS TO CREATE AN ISSUE STATEMENT FOR EACH PROBLEM AREA

Step 1: Review your problem areas and their difficulties. Think about the goal you are trying to achieve in each problem area if these difficulties were to disappear.

Step 2: Create an issue statement question for each problem area. Try a "how can" or "how should" statement first. If this does not seem to fit, move to a "what" question.

Step 3: Check to make sure the question drives exploration of alternatives that, if answered, will resolve the difficulties. Make sure the question is **not** a research question or a yes/no question, and that it does **not** have a judgment or solution in it.

Step 4: Determine if there is an order to the problem areas, meaning one or more of the problem areas have priority over the others because their resolution drives alternatives considered in the subsequent problem areas.

Step 5: Complete the first three columns of the problem area summary table (see Table 7.1 below). List the most important problem area first. Complete the root causes column based on what you know from the stakeholder analysis table and other sources.

TIPS TO CREATE AN ISSUE STATEMENT FOR EACH PROBLEM AREA

- When working as a team on organizational problem solving, focus your team efforts on listing difficulties, grouping them into problem areas, and writing the issue statement for each problem area. This will enhance your team's ability to ask the right questions to resolve the problem, rather than arguing over prematurely identified solutions to fix an undefined problem.

- A well-written issue statement should drive consensus among stakeholders that the question identified is the one that needs answering to resolve the problem.

■ As a student team or a fellow, share your issue statements with your organizational preceptor for feedback.

ISSUE STATEMENT TOOL

As you craft your issue statements, you want to ensure that they accurately capture the key issue in each problem area. And that, in totality, they encompass all of the issues that need resolution to successfully solve the problem.

To support this development and review, summarize your work so far in the problem area summary table as shown in Table 7.1. You can also begin to complete the last column, titled Possible Root Causes, with what you have learned from your stakeholder analysis and other preliminary data. You will come back to this column when you begin the Study phase of the Problem-Solving Method.

Lastly, you will complete the problem statement and the vision for the future in the next substep.

ACTIVITIES TO CREATE ISSUE STATEMENT FOR EACH PROBLEM AREA

Use the difficulties and problem areas you identified in Activities 14 and 15 in Chapter 6 as you work on the Activities that follow.

TABLE 7.1 Problem Area Summary Table

PROBLEM AREA	ISSUE STATEMENT	DIFFICULTIES	POSSIBLE ROOT CAUSES
Problem Statement:			
Vision for the Future:			

■ **DEFINE ACTIVITY 16**

Critique the issue statement for each problem area in the following (i.e., what is wrong with each issue statement?). Remember an issue statement should identify the key issue in the problem area that needs to be answered, and include the barriers and/or context of that issue. In addition, each issue statement should drive consensus among all the stakeholders that it is, in fact, the key question that needs to be addressed to resolve the set of difficulties in the problem area. It should not be a yes/no question or question of fact. It should not have a solution embedded in it.

■ **CRITIQUE THESE ISSUE STATEMENTS**

Goal Misalignment: How can Prism Health System leadership get the stakeholders of the Musculoskeletal Clinical Service Line to understand the importance of reducing the costs of providing care to patients with chronic musculoskeletal issues so that the health system will be the partner of choice for Prism Health Plan's Spine Center of Distinction Program?

Care Model: How can Prism Health System implement the MedSpine joint venture care model in light of the current opposition from many stakeholders affiliated with the Musculoskeletal Clinical Service Line?

Payer Relations: How can Prism Health System reduce its cost of providing care to patients with chronic musculoskeletal issues in light of the reported higher costs and its own health plan's critical viewpoints towards Prism's care for those with neck and back pain?

Decision-Making Process: How can the Musculoskeletal Clinical Service Line dyad leaders ensure they are listening to key stakeholders in light of the opposition to the MedSpine proposal that has been expressed by many of them?

■ **DEFINE ACTIVITY 17**

Rewrite the issue statements for each of the problem areas in Activity 16 so that they reflect the appropriate structure and content of an issue statement.

■ **DEFINE ACTIVITY 18**

How would you reorder the problem areas to show their respective relative importance?

■ **DEFINE ACTIVITY 19**

Complete the first three columns of the problem area summary table in Figure 7.1, listing the problem areas in order of their importance you determined in Activity 18.

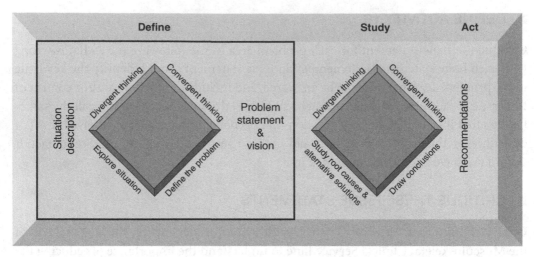

FIGURE 7.2 Completion of the first wave of divergent-convergent thinking.

PRACTICE D3.2: CREATE THE PROBLEM STATEMENT AND VISION FOR THE FUTURE

The issue statements are synthesized into an overall problem statement that summarizes the issue statements, the stakeholders that need to be satisfied by the solution, and the major constraints that must be considered in solving the problem.

The vision for the future is an aspirational statement that articulates the desired outcomes once the problem is solved.

HOW TO CREATE PROBLEM STATEMENT AND VISION FOR THE FUTURE

You now need to write a problem statement that synthesizes and summarizes the key issues across all of the problem areas completely, cogently, and concisely. The constraints and context of the problem areas also need to be articulated in the problem statement, and the key stakeholders who need to be satisfied by the solution need to be identified. It should also take into account any interrelationships in issues that may exist between the problem areas. Problem statements are generally in one or the other formats given in the following.

> *How can (or how should) organization X achieve {stated goals synthesized from across the issue statements} in light of {stated barriers in the issue statements} and/or {broader organizational goals} to the satisfaction of {list of key stakeholders in the situation}?*

> *What is the appropriate {structure, goal, or benchmark} for the organization regarding {key issue(s)}, and how can the organization best achieve that {structure, goal, or benchmark} in light of {stated barriers summarized from across the problem*

areas} and/or {broader organizational goals} to the satisfaction of {list of key stakeholders in the situation}?

When developing a problem statement, try to avoid simply linking each of your issue statements together into one long run-on sentence. Instead, try to summarize the language across the issue statements. Also, when synthesizing the issue statements, be on the lookout for issues that lie at the intersection of problem areas. For example, in The Spinal Frontier case, the lack of agreement on an appropriate care model may be related to the misalignment of goals around the service line.

Once you have written the problem statement, write a brief few sentences about the vision for the future. This vision should articulate the overall aspirational goal that will be achieved by the organization if this problem is successfully resolved. This vision should help answer the "why" for focusing on resolving the problem, and there should be agreement among the stakeholders that this is what the organization should be striving to be.

It is helpful to work as a team to synthesize the issue statements into the problem statement, and to craft the vision for the future. The team needs to reach consensus on both of these outputs for this substep. Similar to the issue statements, this focuses the team's efforts on coming to agreement on asking the right questions, not arguing about solutions. As you gain experience in problem-solving, creating a problem statement and vision for the future that you can clearly articulate will become easier, and you will be able to facilitate a team's problem-solving process.

When you have completed this substep, you have completed the Define phase, and have engaged in the first wave of divergent-convergent thinking of the Problem-Solving Method, as shown in Figure 7.2. You now have the problem areas, issue statements, and a problem statement that help you structure the Study phase of the Problem-Solving Method.

KEY STEPS TO CREATE THE PROBLEM STATEMENT AND VISION FOR THE FUTURE

Step 1: Review your issue statements. Think about the overall goal you are trying to achieve if all of the issue statements are resolved. Look to see if the overall problem lies at the intersection of one or more problem areas

Step 2: Create a problem statement that synthesizes the issue statements or articulates the problem lying at the intersection of two or more problem areas. Try a "how can" or "how should" statement first. If this does not seem to fit, move to a "what" question.

Step 3: List the key stakeholders that need to be satisfied by the solution to the problem.

Step 4: Given the issue statements and the problem statement, write a vision for the future that summarizes the "ought to be" in an aspirational, encompassing way that provides stakeholders with a clear idea of what could be achieved if the problem as stated is solved in its entirety.

TIPS TO CREATE THE PROBLEM STATEMENT AND VISION FOR THE FUTURE

- When working as a team on organizational problem-solving, write the problem statement as a team. This will enhance your team's ability to ask the right questions to resolve the problem, and increase the probability that all relevant stakeholders to the problem have been identified.

- A well-written problem statement should drive consensus among stakeholders that the questions identified are the one that needs answering to resolve the problem.

- As a student team, share your issue statements and the problem statement with your organizational preceptor for feedback.

- Crafting a crisp, clear, cogent problem statement takes practice. You may initially feel that you are engaging in the art of the run-on sentence. But as you become an expert in creating a problem statement, you will be looked upon as an opinion leader in your organization.

PROBLEM STATEMENT AND VISION TOOL

The problem area summary table introduced in Table 7.1 is useful in this substep. Write your problem statement and your vision for the future underneath the table.

ACTIVITIES TO CREATE PROBLEM STATEMENT AND VISION FOR THE FUTURE

■ DEFINE ACTIVITY 20

Which one of the following problem statements best captures, synthesizes, and summarizes the issue statements of The Spinal Frontier? What is wrong with the other problem statements?

Problem Statement #1: What is the optimal care model for patients with chronic neck and back pain that aligns with Prism Health System's Triple Aim goal, in light of the MedSpine joint venture proposal, the high costs of Prism's spine care compared to insurance industry benchmarks, and the health plan's focus on value-based care; and what are the implications of the care model for payer relations and the structure of the service line—to the satisfaction of the Service Line Steering Committee, the Prism Health Plan, patients, and the community?

Problem Statement #2: How can Prism Health System and the Health Plan optimize patient care, achieve a competitive premium rate, and ensure optimal communication/involvement with stakeholders regarding strategic developments, given the MedSpine proposal and the desire to cut costs from the Health Plan, potential layoffs in physical therapy, and disagreements with the spine surgeon, Physical Therapy Director, and the CFO?

Problem Statement #3: How can Prism Health System most effectively be reimbursed for the Musculoskeletal Clinical Service Line services in light of rising hospital care costs, what can the hospital do to ensure proper patient services are rendered within the Musculoskeletal Clinical Service Line, and how can they collaboratively and formally make decisions that help guide the Musculoskeletal Service Line toward the Triple Aim?

■ DEFINE ACTIVITY 21

Which one of the following statements best articulates the vision for the future in the context of the problem? What is wrong with the other statements of the vision for the future?

Vision #1: Prism Health System is a model for integrated care in the Midwest. Prism continuously strives to attain and maintain the Triple Aim of care to ensure that our patients are receiving the most affordable and effective care. Responding to our diverse patient needs and evolving market demand, Prism is committed to refining and adjusting our delivery of care to best match the needs of our patients. We are innovative and willing to press into diverse models of care to ensure that the health of our community is protected and sustained.

Vision #2: A hospital that is recognized by the community for providing top of the line, progressive healthcare with special considerations to the Triple Aim to all patients seeking care. This care can be defined and provided specifically to spine patients in a collaborative effort among the physical therapy, orthopedics, and imaging departments in addition to the Prism Health Plan. Once best practice is established and implemented, the next step will be piloting a bundle payment program.

Vision #3: Prism Health is a highly integrated health system in the Midwest that lives its public commitment of the Triple Aim. We provide high quality and safe patient care, and we are good stewards of our resources by providing cost-effective, affordable care, all while improving the health of our population. In providing these services, we strive to build a culture of collaboration between our health system facilities and our health plan to achieve the Triple Aim.

■ DEFINE ACTIVITY 22

Complete the problem area summary table by putting your problem statement and vision for the future at the bottom of the page.

SUMMARY OF WRITTEN PRODUCTS FROM THE DEFINE PHASE

When you have worked through the Define phase of the Problem-Solving Method in Chapters 5, 6, and 7, you should have completed the following written products from your work:

- Situation Description—both a longer version (about one to three pages) and the Situation and Background sections of an SBAR.
- Consulting Agreement
- Stakeholder Analysis Table
- Problem Area Summary Table (Possible root causes column will be revised in Study step S1)

CHAPTER 8

DEFINE PHASE ACTIVITY KEY

D1.1: DESCRIBE THE SITUATION ACTIVITY KEY (IN CHAPTER 5)

■ **DEFINE ACTIVITY 1 KEY**

Critique the Situation Description

The italicized phrases and the sentences that follow need revising. The number after each phrase or sentence refers to the answer of what is incorrect and what revisions are needed in the rationale following this situation description.

Situation Description

Prism Health System, a highly integrated system in the Midwest that also owns its own health plan, is publicly committed to the Triple Aim. *The Health System needs to reduce the cost of providing care to patients with chronic musculoskeletal issues.* (1) They started a musculoskeletal service line 2 years ago, led by a physician–administrator dyad, to coordinate musculoskeletal care across the continuum. But *their costs are still too high.* (2) Because *the dyad leadership team needs better information to manage the service line,* (3) they were surprised when they were *told that their costs were too high by the health plan CEO.* (4) If Prism Health System can't successfully reduce their costs, *the Prism Health Plan CEO threatened the health system COO* (5) that the health system will not be the preferred partner with the health plan on a Spine Center of Distinction Program.

To reduce costs, Prism Health System is planning to enter into a joint venture with MedSpine, a national provider that specializes in low-cost, high-quality spine care, as documented in peer-reviewed articles. They have received a joint venture proposal from MedSpine, and the Health System COO said that it looks profitable. However, several key stakeholders are not on board with the joint venture, and *the service line leadership has been ignoring their concerns.* (6) *The physician–administrator service line dyad leaders are moving too fast,* (7) and *they aren't engaging in the due diligence required for joint ventures.* (8) *The hospital CFO is opposed because the joint venture will hurt the hospital financially.* (9) *The Director of Physical Therapy is opposed because she will have to lay off staff.* (10) *The Spine Surgeon is not clear why they want to reduce spine surgical volume, since this is what he was hired to do.* (11) He is also upset because the *joint venture hasn't even been discussed with the service line steering committee.* (12) The service line leadership team and the health system COO *need to convince these key stakeholders that a joint venture is the right strategy to pursue to reduce costs.* (13) The health system will also *need to start rewarding its clinical and administrative leaders for value rather than volume and revenue production* to achieve the Triple Aim. (14) (15)

Rationale

(1) Stick to the facts of the case. For example, the Spine Surgeon might not agree that the costs of care need to be reduced. He might say that Prism's patient case mix for musculoskeletal care is more complex than average, resulting in higher costs. At this step, you don't know. It would be a fact to say that the Prism Health Plan CEO desires to reduce the cost of providing care to patients with chronic musculoskeletal issues because its costs are high compared to insurance industry local, regional, and national benchmarks.

(2) Stick to the facts of the case. The case states that Prism Health System's cost of providing spine care is high compared to insurance industry local, regional, and national benchmarks. This does not necessarily mean that costs are "too high." You might uncover reasons during the Study phase of the Problem-Solving Method, for example, the case mix issue mentioned in (1) above, that would justify the current costs incurred by Prism Health System of providing care to patients with chronic musculoskeletal issues.

(3) Stick to the facts of the case. You don't know at this point whether the leadership dyad needs better information. What you do know is that the administrator said his information is incomplete, and he cited volume, utilization, and revenue data. He did not mention any cost data. This should clue you in that a *possible root cause* is that the leadership team needs more relevant, timely, complete, and accurate cost data. *But surmising about root causes does not belong in the situation description.* It is a fact to say in the situation description that the administrator said his data to track performance is incomplete, and he did not cite cost data, but that the volume, utilization, and revenue data were either on track or trending upward as desired.

(4) Stick to the facts of the case. The Prism Health Plan CEO stated that the cost of providing spine care for Prism Health System patients is high compared to the insurance industry's local, regional, and national benchmarks, and is rising rapidly. This is making it difficult to price the Prism Health Plan's products at a competitive premium rate. He did not specifically say that the costs were "too high." Always state the difficulty as it was said to keep it as factual to the original statement as possible. It would be difficult for stakeholders who do not believe the costs are "too high" to argue with the fact that the costs are high compared to insurance industry standards

(5)   Stick to the facts of the case. The Prism Health System COO did not say that the Health Plan CEO threatened him. Avoid value-laden words like "threatened" that evoke negative emotion, especially when that wasn't what was said. Even if that was something that the COO said, it is generally not helpful to phrase it like that when writing the situation description, unless it is absolutely germane to the problem. It would be better to say: If Prism Health System can't successfully reduce their costs, they risk not being the preferred partner with the health plan on a Spine Center of Distinction Program.

(6)   This is an opinion of several key stakeholders, and needs to be stated as such. It would be better to state it as: "Several key stakeholders expressed that they feel their concerns about the joint venture are not being heard by the Prism Health System leadership." This makes the sentence a fact.

(7)   Stick to the facts of the case. No one in the case said the leadership team was moving too fast. If this is an opinion or inference of one of the student team members, it should not be in the situation description. Instead, you could be more specific and factual about the timeline. For example: "Within the past 2 months, the leadership team has researched MedSpine's quality, costs, and outcomes, and met with MedSpine. Following that one meeting, MedSpine provided Prism Health System with a joint venture proposal, which the service line leaders and COO are planning to accept and implement."

(8)   Stick to the facts of the case. No one in the case said the leadership team is not engaging in the due diligence required for joint ventures. If this is an opinion or inference of one of the student team members, it should not be in the situation description.

(9)   This is a stakeholder's opinion, and is stated as such: "The hospital CFO is opposed to the joint venture because she believes it will hurt the hospital financially." But, remember to keep what is told to you by stakeholders in confidence for a situation description shared with the organization. See the suggested sentence in (11).

(10) This is a stakeholder's opinion, and is stated as such: "The Physical Therapy Director is opposed to the joint venture because she believes she will have to lay off staff." But, remember to keep what is told to you by stakeholders in confidence for a situation description shared with the organization. See the suggested sentence in (11).

(11) This is not what the spine surgeon said. Be sure to accurately capture what was said. Don't make inferences about stakeholders' comments that aren't accurate. For example, the following is a fact: "The Spine Surgeon was surprised about the proposed joint venture, because he thought he was successfully building the spine surgery program." A way to reword sentences in (9), (10), and (11) in the situation description shared with the organization might be: "Several stakeholders expressed concerns about the negative

impacts they believe the joint venture might have on the hospital and patients, including staff layoffs, financial implications to the hospital, and clinical quality of spine care."

(12)   It is unknown whether this is a fact. It was stated as such by one stakeholder, but it would require verification through further research. However, several did report that they have not been involved in the joint venture discussions. Since the Steering Committee meets quarterly, and the Administrative dyad leader said he met with the Prism Health Plan CEO "a couple of months ago," it is possible that the joint venture has not been discussed at these meetings. The sentence could be revised as follows to make it a fact: "One stakeholder stated that the joint venture has not been discussed at the last Service Line Steering Committee meeting."

(13)   *This is a solution.* And, if this is an opinion or inference of one of the student team members, it should not be in the situation description.

(14)   Stick to the facts of the case. This sentence could be a *potential alternative solution. Potential alternative solutions do not belong in the situation description.*

(15)   Several relevant difficulties are missing from the situation description. These difficulties must be included because otherwise they will not be investigated for possible resolution when solving the problem, and you will have committed a Type III error. The situation description omits information about the services included in the service line, the composition and purpose of the service line steering committee, and the current reporting relationships. These all need further exploration. The situation does not mention that the health plan CEO raised the cost issue several months prior to when it came up again most recently, but the administrator of the service line did not follow up at that time. The Director of Physical Therapy mentioned that the hospital does not have protocols for managing patients with chronic neck and back pain. The stakeholders interviewed also report that they haven't been involved in the joint venture discussions, although two of them are on the service line steering committee.

■ DEFINE ACTIVITY 2 KEY

A sample situation description follows.

Sample Situation Description

Prism Health System, a highly integrated system in the Midwest that also owns its own health plan, is publicly committed to the Triple Aim. It wants to be recognized as the provider of choice by the community for spine care. Two years ago, they started a Musculoskeletal Clinical Service Line to coordinate program development across the system for its patients with spine problems, such as chronic neck and back pain. They recently hired a new Spine Surgeon, Dr. Grant Norton, to build a spine surgery program, and it was reported at the kickoff meeting that this has been progressing well. They also have a thriving orthopedics program.

The service line is managed using a dyad partner model comprised of a physician and an administrator. The clinical dyad leader is an orthopedic surgeon, and reports to the chair of the Orthopedics department. The administrator dyad leader graduated with his MHA degree 5 years ago, and has been in this position for about a year. The Physical and Occupational Therapy Directors also report to him. He reports to the Prism Health System COO. The specialities in the Musculoskeletal Service Line include Orthopedics, Sports Medicine, and a nonsurgical program, Rheumatology. Each of these specialties also has a dyad leadership model.

The Musculoskeletal Clinical Service Line Steering Committee provides input into decisions about the service line, but doesn't have formal voting authority. It meets quarterly, and is comprised of the service line clinical and administrator dyad leaders, the recently hired spine surgeon, the Health System COO, the Health Plan CEO, the hospital CFO, and the chair of the Orthopedics department. It is chaired by the clinical dyad leader and the Orthopedics chair.

Approximately 5 to 6 months ago, the health plan CEO encouraged the administrator service line leader to talk with MedSpine. The administrator did not do so until the health plan CEO told him about 2 months ago that Prism Health System's costs of providing spine care are high compared to insurance industry local, regional, and national benchmarks, and are rising rapidly. The health plan CEO said this is making it difficult to price the Prism Health Plan's products at a competitive premium rate.

This was a surprise to the service line dyad leaders, as their internal data, which the administrator leader said was incomplete, nevertheless showed that the service line efforts were on track for revenue and utilization, and that physical therapy, musculoskeletal imaging, and surgical volumes had been trending upward as desired. The health plan CEO also told the health system COO that they are planning to start a Spine Center of Distinction Program that is based on outcomes and costs, and they would like to pilot bundled payments with the "right partner." The health plan CEO indicated that Prism Health System is not guaranteed to be that partner because it needs to improve its ability to provide value-based spine care.

At that meeting 2 months ago, the Health Plan CEO strongly encouraged the service line leaders to meet with MedSpine, a national company that specializes in spine care. MedSpine provides non-surgical spine care. The group, which was founded by an orthopedic surgeon and an exercise physiologist, is a provider of non-surgical, intensive exercise and strengthening based care to patients with chronic neck and back pain. The service line leaders researched MedSpine, and said that published reports of their costs, quality and outcomes are favorable.

The administrator service line leader recently met with MedSpine. Shortly thereafter, the MedSpine leadership team sent the health system an initial proposal to form a joint venture to own and operate a MedSpine program at Prism Health System. The Health

System COO reports that their initial vetting of the MedSpine proposal is that it looks good and that he finds it promising. He said it appears profitable, it is clinically efficient with high quality providers, the Health Plan sees value in the organization, and the attorney says the contract looks good. He and the service line leaders plan to move forward on the joint venture as they say it will position Prism Health System well given its commitment to the Triple Aim.

The administrator service line leader mentioned that there has been some pushback from some people in the hospital. The students' subsequent conversations with the director of Physical Therapy, the hospital CFO, and the spine surgeon revealed their misgivings about the joint venture. They reported that they had not been involved in the discussions, and one of them reported that the joint venture had not been discussed at the steering committee meetings.

Other concerns expressed by one or more of them are that the joint venture is not a good decision because the spine surgery program is successful; MedSpine's treatment approach is not good for patients; Prism should not bring in an outside organization when Prism doesn't have its own care protocols for managing patients with chronic neck and back pain; the Physical Therapy department will have to lay off staff; the hospital's revenue, operating margins, and surgeons will be hurt because of reduced spine surgery and imaging volumes; and the health plan should not be telling the delivery system how to provide care.

■ DEFINE ACTIVITY 3 KEY

Example SBAR

The Situation and Background of the SBAR tool is a brief summary format of the situation description. An example Situation and Background summary for an SBAR tool is shown in Exhibit 8.1.

■ DEFINE ACTIVITY 4 KEY

Student Team Meeting With Faculty Advisor

One approach is for the students to share their written situation description with the faculty advisor during a meeting for discussion. Based on what the students have learned, it appears that the scope for the project should be either changed or expanded beyond an implementation plan for the MedSpine joint venture.

The goal for the meeting with the faculty advisor should be to develop an action plan for circling back with the organizational preceptors to discuss what the student team has learned, and to gain consensus that the student project should move forward with a scope that focuses more broadly on what is the appropriate care model for patients with chronic back and neck problems, as opposed to focus solely on how to implement the joint venture proposal.

The students should take the lead in contacting their Prism preceptors, with the faculty advisor included in any email correspondence. They should request a follow-up meeting with the organizational preceptors to discuss the project and its scope.

EXHIBIT 8.1

COMPLETED SITUATION AND BACKGROUND IN SBAR

S	Situation	Prism Health System's costs of providing care for patients with chronic neck and back problems are high compared to insurance industry local, regional, and national benchmarks, and continue to rise. The Prism Health Plan CEO has indicated that this makes it difficult to price the premium rates competitively for Prism's spine care. To reduce costs while maintaining quality of providing care, several Prism Health System leaders plan to enter into a joint venture with MedSpine, a national provider of spine care that provides non-surgical treatment for chronic back problems. However, other hospital stakeholders do not agree with this decision, as they believe it will not be in the hospital's best interest for a variety of reasons.
B	Background	Prism Health System, a highly integrated system in the Midwest that also owns its own health plan, is publicly committed to the Triple Aim and wants to be recognized as the provider of choice by the community for spine care. Their Musculoskeletal Service Line's volume and revenue have been increasing under the leadership of the recently hired spine surgeon. The increasing volume and revenue of the Musculoskeletal Service Line is beneficial for the hospital, but not for the health plan.

■ **DEFINE ACTIVITY 5 KEY**

Understanding the Context of the Project

Following are example questions that could be researched by the student team prior to the kickoff meeting to better understand the context of the project.

- ■ What is the Triple Aim, and what challenges does it present to healthcare organizations who are trying to achieve its goals?
- ■ What are service lines, what are their goals, and how are they typically structured?
- ■ What are considered best practices in the clinical management of patients with chronic musculoskeletal conditions?
- ■ What are the challenges faced by healthcare organizations that also have their own health plans?

D1.2: SCOPE THE WORK ACTIVITY KEY (IN CHAPTER 5)

■ **DEFINE ACTIVITY 6 KEY**

Revised Summary of Project Deliverable

The project deliverable should not have a predetermined solution (e.g., do the joint venture) embedded in it. Focus on delivering a product that helps the organization achieve their stated goal given the current organizational context of why that goal is important. For example, the deliverable given in the following expands the deliverable beyond focusing only on a joint venture:

Our project team will develop recommendations and an implementation plan for a care model that best supports Prism Health System's goal of being the provider of choice by the community for spine care, given their commitment to the Triple Aim, the MedSpine joint venture opportunity, and recognizing that their current costs of providing spine care are rising and are high compared to insurance industry local, regional, and national benchmarks.

■ DEFINE ACTIVITY 7 KEY

Role Play Follow-Up Meeting

The goal for your follow-up meeting with Prism Health System should focus on changing the scope from implementing a predetermined solution to one that will identify and study a range of potential alternative care models that will help them achieve their goals of being the provider of choice for spine care while achieving the Triple Aim.

To achieve your goal for the meeting, your team will need to think about how to share what you have learned in your initial meetings with stakeholders in a factual manner, as well as mention some of the other issues that may need investigation, such as reporting structures in the service line, and how to address the opposition by some key stakeholders to the joint venture.

Be respectful and be factual.

■ DEFINE ACTIVITY 8 KEY

Complete a Project Consulting Agreement

Some pointers as you complete your project consulting agreement:

- For the Project Scope item, in thinking about the departments to include in your research as you conduct your project, the Musculoskeletal Clinical Service Line, the Orthopedics Department, MedSpine, and the Health Plan should be at the top of your mind But, remember to include the Physical Therapy and Rehab Departments, even though they are not currently part of the Service Line. They would figure prominently in models of care for chronic back pain. The key processes to study would be the flow paths across the continuum of care for patients with chronic back pain.
- For the Approach, be sure to be clear about getting copies of the data, reports, and other documents you have already learned about in these first meetings of your project. These include the data held by the health plan regarding Prism's costs of spine care and the benchmarks. From Prism Health System, the data the Musculoskeletal Clinical Service Line administrator mentioned in the kickoff meeting, and finding out if the health system tracks cost and outcomes data for the service line, and whether it is readily available for the service line

leaders. You should also ask for copies of the published MedSpine articles mentioned in the kickoff meeting so that you can read them to gain better contextual knowledge about their clinical model of spine care.

D2.1 BEGIN: STAKEHOLDER ANALYSIS ACTIVITY KEY (IN CHAPTER 6)

■ DEFINE ACTIVITY 9 KEY

As shown in Table 8.1, there are many stakeholders in this situation that should potentially be interviewed by the student team. Some stakeholders are mentioned only by role

TABLE 8.1 The Spinal Frontier Stakeholders and Roles

STAKEHOLDER NAME	STAKEHOLDER ROLE
Anthony Hayden	MCSL Administrator Dyad Leader and Service Line Steering Committee Member; Manager of Physical Therapy and Occupational Therapy Directors
Dr. LaTonya Waters	MCSL Clinical Dyad Leader and Co-Chair of the MCSL Steering Committee
Dr. Diwakar Patel	Chair of Orthopedics and Co-Chair of the MCSL Steering Committee; Manager of Dr. LaTonya Waters
Charles Dressen	Prism Health System COO and MCSL Steering Committee Member; Manager of Anthony Hayden
Dr. Grant Norton	New Spine Surgeon and MCSL Steering Committee Member
Nadeem Aziz	Prism Health Plan CEO and MCSL Steering Committee Member
Sarah Wallace	Hospital CFO and MCSL Steering Committee Member
Andrea Meyer	Physical Therapy Director (not part of MCSL or Steering Committee)
?	Occupational Therapy Director (not part of MCSL or Steering Committee)
?	Orthopedics Dyad Leaders (part of MCSL)
?	Sports Medicine Dyad Leaders (part of MCSL)
?	Rheumatology Dyad Leaders (part of MCSL)
?	MedSpine Leadership Team
?	Prism Health System Attorney
?	Prism Health System CEO
?	Prism Health System Board of Directors
?	Prism Health Plan Board of Directors
	Patients (and their families) with chronic neck and back pain treated by MCSL
	Community served by Prism Health System and Prism Health Plan

MCSL, musculoskeletal clinical service line.

in the case. It is always helpful to ask for organizational charts as part of the stakeholder interviews (see question 28 of the Interview Guide Tool, Exhibit 6.1 in Chapter 6) to help identify potential interviewees based on the situation.

Remember that the system leadership, including the CEO and the Board, are always stakeholders. This doesn't mean that they will be interviewed for every problem that needs resolution in the organization. But you should always keep their point of view in mind as you work through the Problem-Solving Method. Also, remember that patients, their families, and the community served are always stakeholders.

■ DEFINE ACTIVITY 10 KEY

Based on what you know from the case, summarize each stakeholder's point of view in the stakeholder analysis table. Each stakeholder should be recorded in their own row in the table. Remember that statements in the stakeholder analysis table are perceptions and opinions; they are not facts. An example is provided for Sarah Wallace, the hospital CFO, in Table 8.2. But you should complete the stakeholder analysis table for as many of the stakeholders in Table 8.1 as possible at this phase of the Problem-Solving Method.

When you have completed the stakeholder analysis table for all stakeholders, you should pay attention to where there are differences in perceptions and opinions. For example, you can see that Ms. Wallace's perceptions of success are driven by a hospital volume and revenue production view. If you look at Dr. Norton's comments, you can see that he also perceives success as driven by volume of procedures.

But Prism Health System is striving to achieve the Triple Aim, which means focusing on value (outcomes and costs of care), not just volume. A value view of success is held by the Prism Health Plan CEO and, increasingly, Prism Health System's CEO, COO, and the MCSL dyad leaders. Thus, there is a misalignment of goals across the stakeholders that needs to be addressed.

■ DEFINE ACTIVITY 11 KEY

Interview Guide Questions by Stakeholder

Dyad Leadership Team Questions

The Dyad Leadership Team of the Musculoskeletal Clinical Service Line (MCSL) should be asked all of the questions in the Prism Health System and MCSL section of the interview guide (questions 1 through 19). However, they may not be engaged in payer negotiations, and might tell you that they can't answer questions 18 and 19. You should also ask them for organizational charts of Prism Health System and the Service Line (question 28) and the remainder of the General questions at the end of the interview guide (questions 29–31).

Director of Physical Therapy Questions

The Director of Physical Therapy is not part of the MCSL, although she reports to Anthony Hayden. However, her department would have interactions with at least some

TABLE 8.2 Stakeholder Analysis Table

STAKEHOLDER	GOAL	PERCEIVED DIFFICULTIES	PERCEIVED ROOT CAUSES (WHY?)	SUGGESTED ALTERNATIVE SOLUTIONS	ADDITIONAL INSIGHTS PROVIDED
Sarah Wallace, hospital CFO	A financially healthy hospital Rewarded in performance evaluations and salaries for contributing to the financial well-being of the hospital	MedSpine joint venture is a terrible solution. It will reduce spine surgery and imaging volume, which will hurt surgeons, physial therapy, and the hospital's revenue and operating margin Health Plan is telling Health System how it should provide care	Hospital revenue and incentive structure are driven by surgical and imaging volume MCSL leaders are listening to the Prism Health Plan CEO, not the r own clinicians	Don't engage in MedSpine joint venture Focus on activities that will generate increasing volume and revenue for the hospital	She has volume and financial data for the MCSL

MCSL, musculoskeletal clinical service line.
(Row completed for Sarah Wallace, Hospital CFO.)

of the patients in the MCSL. Thus, she should be asked a subset of the questions in the Prism Health System and MCSL section of the interview guide. The ones most relevant to her would likely be questions 1, 2, 7, 9, and 10. In addition, all stakeholders interviewed should be asked the general questions 29 to 31.

Example of Additional Questions Not in Interview Guide

Often, the additional questions that need to be asked flow as probing follow-up questions based on how the stakeholder is answering a question. This is what is meant by asking probing questions to clarify what the stakeholder is saying. For example, the student team learned at the kickoff meeting that the Administrator Dyad Leader mentioned volume data, but not cost data. It would be helpful to ask him what type of data he is provided regularly regarding the MCSL, and what type of data he wished he received.

Then, when meeting with the hospital CFO, the students could ask whether the type of data the Administrator Dyad Leader wished he received is available, but just not provided to him as a standing report. This would help the student team be more specific about the facts regarding data available to manage the MCSL. But, at this point in time, data issues remain unclear. It will need to be further researched in the Study phase of the Problem-Solving Method.

The Director of Physical Therapy mentioned that Prism Health System does not have protocols for managing patients with chronic neck and back pain. This should be probed for more information. What should be included in these protocols? Is there a reason that Prism Health System may not have protocols? Is there a professional physical therapy national organization that she recommends the students talk with or review their website to learn more about best practices in such protocols?

■ DEFINE ACTIVITY 12 KEY

If there are differences in perceptions among the stakeholders, it is important to try to study the stakeholder analysis to understand the reasons for those differences. Are there differences in goals or values? In knowledge of the context in which the situation resides? In knowledge or use of the facts? In preferred solutions?

These differences provide you with insights as to whether there are particular data that are critical to uncover during the Study phase, especially with respect to root causes and how various alternative solutions address the issues identified in the problem areas.

They also help you understand what decision criteria are most relevant to different stakeholders when choosing among alternatives, and how they might be weighing those criteria differently.

It also helps you understand which stakeholders might oppose different alternatives, and get you to start thinking early on in the Study phase about a communications plan to address this opposition.

Remember that successful resolution of the problem requires successful implementation of well-studied solutions. You need to ensure that the final set of solutions you recommend are acceptable to the stakeholders involved. The solutions might not be the ones that were preferred by certain stakeholder groups, but your stakeholder analysis should help you develop a communication strategy to build consensus for a course of action that will ultimately be viewed as acceptable to all the stakeholders involved.

D2.2: IDENTIFY DIFFICULTIES ACTIVITY KEY (IN CHAPTER 6)

■ **DEFINE ACTIVITY 13 KEY**

Each statement provides an answer as to whether it is a difficulty, and, if not, why.

1. Prism Health System needs to reduce the cost of providing care to patients with chronic musculoskeletal care needs. *This is not a difficulty, as it is not a fact. It is an opinion of some of the stakeholders. The fact is that Prism Health System's costs of providing care to patients with chronic neck and back pain is high compared to insurance industry local, regional, and national benchmarks, and continue to rise. It helps to state the fact in this manner so that those who are opposed to the joint venture understand the fact based on data, not the opinions of those who think the costs are too high.*

2. Health Plan CEO indicates Prism costs for patients with chronic musculoskeletal care needs are high compared to insurance industry benchmarks. *This is a difficulty, as it is a fact.*

3. The MedSpine proposal will financially harm the hospital because it will result in layoffs and decreased revenues. *This is not a difficulty, as it is not a fact. It is an opinion of some of the stakeholders. To make it a difficulty, it needs to state that some stakeholders believe this to be true.*

4. The Administrative Dyad Partner of the Musculoskeletal Clinical Service Line was surprised when told by the Health Plan CEO that their costs of care were higher than industry benchmarks. *This is a difficulty, as it is a fact.*

5. The Health Plan CEO is overstepping his bounds when telling the Health System to talk with MedSpine. *This is not a difficulty, as it is not a fact. It is an opinion of one of the stakeholders. To make it a difficulty, it needs to state that a stakeholder believes this to be true.*

6. The organization needs to look at all their data before deciding what to do. *This is not a difficulty, as it is not a fact. This statement describes a process of reviewing data during research.*

7. Some stakeholders view increasing utilization for musculoskeletal services as a success, while others perceive that as a problem given Prism's commitment to the Triple Aim. *This is a difficulty, as it is a fact. The health plan CEO sees increasing utilization as increasing costs of care, while many in the hospital view increased utilization as revenue for the hospital.*

8. The hospital does not have protocols for managing patients with musculo-skeletal issues. *This is not a difficulty, as it is not a fact. You don't have enough information at this time to know whether or not this is a fact, as it is a statement made by one stakeholder. You will need to conduct research during the Study phase to determine if this statement is verifiable as true. It needs to be rewritten to make it a difficulty—state that someone said this to make it a difficulty.*

9. Hospital CFO believes that the MedSpine proposal will hurt the hospital financially. *This is a difficulty, as it identifies that this stakeholder feels this is true.*

10. The Physical Therapy Department should be part of the Musculoskeletal Clinical Service Line to improve continuity of care. *This is not a difficulty, as it is not a fact. It is assuming an alternative solution. Alternative solutions are not difficulties.*

11. Many stakeholders feel that the administrator of the Musculoskeletal Clinical Service Line is not listening to them. *This is a difficulty, as it identifies that many stakeholders feel this is true.*

12. This major strategic MedSpine joint venture decision was made outside of the committee structure that is intended to provide input into the Musculoskeletal Clinical Service Line. *This is not a difficulty, as it is not a fact. You don't have enough information at this time to know whether or not this is a fact, as it is a statement made by one stakeholder. You will need to conduct research during the Study phase to determine if this statement is verifiable as true. It should be included as a difficulty by indicating that someone said this is what happened.*

13. The organization needs better spreadsheets and data to track their costs of care. *This is not a difficulty, as it is not a fact. It is assuming an alternative solution. Alternative solutions are not difficulties.*

14. The Musculoskeletal Clinical Service Line administrator didn't know Prism treatment costs were higher than industry standards until told by the Health Plan CEO. *This is a difficulty, as it is stated in the case as a fact.*

15. The Health Plan CEO is telling Prism Health System how to provide clinical care. *This is not a difficulty, as it is not a fact. It is an opinion of one of the stakeholders. To make it a difficulty, it needs to state that a stakeholder believes this to be true.*

16. Prism Health System is not acting like a value-based health system and will be unsuccessful in achieving the Triple Aim. *This is not a difficulty, as it is not a fact. It is an opinion of one of the stakeholders. To make it a difficulty, it needs to state that a stakeholder believes this to be true.*

17. Musculoskeletal Clinical Service Line dyad leaders are not listening to their clinical and financial stakeholders. *This is not a difficulty, as it is not a fact. It is an opinion of one of the stakeholders. To make it a difficulty, it needs to state that a stakeholder believes this to be true.*

18. The stakeholders opposed to the MedSpine proposal don't understand the importance of value-based care to succeed in today's marketplace. *This is not a difficulty, as it is not a fact. You don't have enough information at this time to know whether or not this is a fact. It is a possible root cause for the disagreement about pursuing the joint venture.*

19. Prism Health System should partner with MedSpine to remain competitive in the marketplace. *This is not a difficulty, as it is not a fact. It is assuming an alternative solution. Alternative solutions are not difficulties.*

20. Prism Health system should not partner with MedSpine because of the opposition to the strategic partnership proposal. *This is not a difficulty, as it is not a fact. It is assuming an alternative solution. Alternative solutions are not difficulties.*

■ DEFINE ACTIVITY 14 KEY

The following are difficulties:

1. There are multiple reporting relationships of members in the service line. The service line administrator leader reports to the health system COO, the service line clinician leader reports to the Orthopedics department chair, and several departments in the service line have their own dyad leadership structures.

2. The role of the Service Line Steering Committee in the MedSpine joint venture decision is unclear. The decision to accept the MedSpine joint venture's proposal was made within the past couple of months, and the spine surgeon reported that it was not discussed with the committee.

3. Several stakeholders report being unhappy with the MedSpine joint venture decision-making process. They feel that they weren't involved in the decision and that their concerns are not being listened to.

4. The administrator service line leader mentioned that there has been some pushback from some people in the hospital regarding the proposed MedSpine joint venture, but has been moving forward with the proposal.

5. Several stakeholders are opposed to the MedSpine joint venture solution. They believe it will hurt the hospital's volume and revenue, hurt the physical therapy department because of layoffs, and hurt the surgeons. The hospital CFO believes the service line leaders are jumping to a "terrible solution."

6. The health plan CEO encouraged the service line administrator to talk with MedSpine several months ago, but the administrator neglected to do so until learning that their costs for spine care are high compared to insurance industry benchmarks.

7. Prism Health System's costs of providing spine care are high compared to insurance industry local, regional and national benchmarks, and are rising rapidly. The health plan CEO said this is making it difficult to price the Prism Health Plan's products at a competitive premium rate.

8. The health plan CEO said that they will be starting a Spine Center of Distinction Program, and that the Prism Health System risks not being the "right partner" for their value-based initiative that will be based on costs and outcomes of spine care.

9. The musculoskeletal service line leaders were surprised when they learned that their costs of spine care are high compared to insurance industry benchmarks.

10. The administrator reported that their internal data are incomplete, but that the service line was on track and trending upward as desired for revenue, volume, and utilization in PT, musculoskeletal imaging, and surgical procedures. He did not mention cost data for the service line.

11. Prism Health System's current care model focuses on volume and revenue of services provided. This does not align with their commitment to the Triple Aim.

12. The newly hired spine surgeon is not convinced that the MedSpine care model is good for patients.

13. The newly hired spine surgeon does not think the joint venture is needed because he has been successfully building the spine surgery program, as evidenced by increasing volume and revenues.

14. The physical therapist is opposed to bringing outsiders in to provide care, especially since she reports that Prism Health System doesn't have any protocols in place to manage patients with chronic neck and back pain.

15. The hospital CFO says that they should be deciding the clinical care model, not the health plan.

D2.3: PROBLEM AREAS ACTIVITY KEY (IN CHAPTER 6)

■ DEFINE ACTIVITY 15 KEY

There are no right or wrong answers in grouping the difficulties into problem areas, but the groupings should be as mutually exclusive of each other as possible. Some of the difficulties can fit logically into more than one bucket. Each bucket of difficulties should represent a common theme that helps name that problem area.

Grouping the 15 numbered difficulties in the Activity 14 key given previously, example buckets could be the four listed below.

BUCKET	A	B	C	D
DIFFICULTIES	# 5, 7, 8, 9, 10, 12, 14, 15	# 7, 8	# 1, 2, 3, 4, 6, 9, 15	# 5, 11, 13

Then, looking at the themes of the difficulties in the four buckets, the problem area names that capture the theme of the difficulties in the buckets could be:

PROBLEM AREA NAME	CARE MODEL	PAYER RELATIONS	DECISION MAKING PROCESS	GOAL MISALIGNMENT
Bucket	A	B	C	D

D3.1: CREATE ISSUE STATEMENTS ACTIVITY KEY (IN CHAPTER 7)

■ DEFINE ACTIVITY 16 KEY

Critique Each Issue Statement

Goal Misalignment: How can Prism Health System leadership get the stakeholders of the Musculoskeletal Clinical Service Line to understand the importance of reducing the costs of providing care to patients with chronic musculoskeletal issues so that the health system will be the partner of choice for Prism Health Plan's Spine Center of Distinction Program?

This issue statement makes an assumption that the stakeholders don't understand the importance of reducing costs of care. It also assumes a solution of becoming the health plan's partner for the Spine Center of Distinction Program. This issue statement would not garner support of all stakeholders as written.

Care Model: How can Prism Health System implement the MedSpine joint venture care model in light of the current opposition from many stakeholders affiliated with the Musculoskeletal Clinical Service Line?

This issue statement assumes a solution of implementing the MedSpine joint venture. This issue statement would not garner support of all stakeholders as written.

Payer Relations: How can Prism Health System reduce its costs of providing care to patients with chronic musculoskeletal issues in light of the reported higher costs and its own health plan critical viewpoints toward Prism's care of those with neck and back pain?

This issue statement assumes a goal of reducing the cost of providing care, when you know from writing the difficulties that this is not a difficulty as stated. Also, it is not helpful to frame the health plan as having critical viewpoints of the health system. Find a more productive way to state that the health plan has some concerns. This issue statement would not garner support of all stakeholders as written.

Decision-Making Process: How can the Musculoskeletal Clinical Service Line dyad leaders ensure they are listening to key stakeholders in light of the opposition to the MedSpine proposal that has been expressed by many of them?

This issue statement assumes a solution—get the dyad leaders to listen better. This is a very narrow approach for how one might improve the decision-making process. An issue statement should never have a solution embedded in it.

■ DEFINE ACTIVITY 17 KEY

Example issue statements follow. You can see that without reading the situation description, you have a pretty complete idea of what is in it by reading the issue statements. The statements capture the detail of the difficulties.

Goal Misalignment: How can Prism Health System align the goals of its Musculoskeletal Clinical Service Line to its commitment to the Triple Aim, in light of Prism's high costs of spine care compared to insurance industry benchmarks, and the Service Line's reliance on volume, activity, and revenue data to judge the success of the service line?

Care Model: What is the optimal care model for treating chronic neck and back pain, in light of the MedSpine joint venture proposal and resistance to it by some key stakeholders, Prism's high costs of providing spine care compared to insurance industry benchmarks, and the health plan's increasing focus on value-based care for the health system's Triple Aim goal?

Payer Relations: How can the Prism Health System best leverage the expertise and resources of its health plan to achieve the Triple Aim, given that the health plan's CEO has expressed concerns about the health system's ability to provide value-based care?

Decision-Making Process: What is the appropriate decision-making process for the Musculoskeletal Clinical Service Line, in light of the current composition, leadership, operating, and authority structure of its Steering Committee, and the concerns expressed by several key stakeholders on the Committee that they have not had input into the MedSpine joint venture?

■ DEFINE ACTIVITY 18 KEY

The problem list should be ordered with the Care Model problem area as the primary issue. This is because it is the main issue that needs resolution. Also, the care model solution recommended for this problem area will likely affect the recommended solutions for the other problem areas.

If, in conducting your research, you find that the mechanisms to align goals depends on how the health system engages with the health plan, then the Payer Relations problem area would be next. Then, third would be the Goal Misalignment problem area. The final problem area of the Decision-Making Process would flow from the first three problem areas.

Thus, the problem list in priority order is: (1) Care Model; (2) Payer Relations; (3) Goal Misalignment; and (4) Decision-Making Process. This is the order in which you would list them in your problem area summary table.

■ **DEFINE ACTIVITY 19 KEY**

The Care Model problem area has been completed in Table 8.3. Your answer should include all of the problem areas. They should be listed in priority order in the table. The Possible Root Causes column should remain blank for now.

D3.2: CREATE PROBLEM STATEMENT ACTIVITY KEY (IN CHAPTER 7)

■ **DEFINE ACTIVITY 20 KEY**

Problem statement #1 best synthesizes the key issues, the goals, the barriers, and the context of the problem. It also best articulates the stakeholders.

Problem statement #2 is too vague. If you hadn't read the situation description, you would have no idea that the patient care in question focuses on treating chronic neck and back pain. It doesn't articulate the interests of the health plan for value-based care. It assumes a solution of needing improved communication. It doesn't state whose desire it is to reduce costs, nor who believes there will be potential layoffs, so it states two opinions, which are not difficulties. It ends by focusing on the negative aspects of disagreement. It neglects to list the key stakeholders who must be satisfied by the solution. This is not a problem statement that is likely to get all of the key stakeholders to agree that this is the question that needs to be answered to solve the problem.

TABLE 8.3 Problem Area Summary Table

PROBLEM AREA	ISSUE STATEMENT	DIFFICULTIES*	POSSIBLE ROOT CAUSES
Care Model	What is the optimal care model for treating chronic neck and back pain, in light of the MedSpine joint venture proposal and resistance to it by some key stakeholders, Prism's high costs of providing spine care, the health plan's increasing focus on value-based care, and the health system's Triple Aim goal?	5, 7, 8, 10, 12, 14, 15	

*See numbered list of difficulties in Chapter 8, Activity 14.
(Completed for the Care Model problem area.)

Problem Statement: (To be completed in Define Activity 22.)

Vision for the Future: (To be completed in Define Activity 22.)

Problem statement #3 is totally off base. It missed the boat. It leads with how to get reimbursed, which isn't part of the situation description at all. It says that hospital care costs are going up, which also isn't what the difficulty says. What we do know for a fact is that the spine care costs are high compared to insurance industry benchmarks, and have been rising. But this does not mean that hospital care costs are increasing.

Using the words "what can the hospital do to ensure proper patient services are rendered within the Musculoskeletal Clinical Service Line" will likely make many of the key stakeholders angry, as it implies that proper patient services are not being provided. It assumes a solution of collaborative and formal decision-making. Avoid wording that appears to place blame or can be interpreted as being denigrating to one or more stakeholder groups.

And finally, the issue statements as written do not list the key stakeholders that need to be satisfied by the solution to the problem.

This problem statement will likely create anger and disagreement—the exact opposite of what a problem statement needs to achieve.

■ DEFINE ACTIVITY 21 KEY

Vision #3 is the most effective vision statement given the problem being solved. It leads with a statement of being highly integrated and publicly committed to the Triple Aim. It then describes what that means in terms of cost, quality, and outcomes of care. It ends by articulating a desired culture of collaboration between Prism's health system and health plan to achieve the Triple Aim goal.

Vision #2 is ineffective, inaccurate, and uninspiring. It starts by focusing on the hospital, not the fact that Prism is now a health system. It focuses on collaboration within the hospital walls between departments, a very micro level view. It ends with tactical level goals—establishing and implementing best practices (vague) and piloting bundled payments. In summary, vision statements should be aspirational. This one is not.

Vision #1 is better than Vision #2, but it still lacks aspirational vision. It is generic and vague. And, given the more recent addition of the health plan to Prism, it totally ignores that the health plan exists, and that this provides an opportunity to collaborate to achieve the Triple Aim. Overall, this is a statement that seems like it has strung together healthcare buzzwords, but it doesn't inspire or aspire.

■ DEFINE ACTIVITY 22 KEY

You end the Define phase by adding your problem statement and vision for the future to the problem area summary table. For example, you would add the following to Table 8.3.

Problem Statement: What is the optimal care model for patients with chronic neck and back pain that aligns with Prism Health System's Triple Aim goal, in light of the Med-Spine joint venture proposal, the high costs of Prism's spine care, and the health plan's focus on value-based care; and what are the implications of the care model for payer relations and the decision-making structure of the service line—to the satisfaction of the Service Line Steering Committee, the Prism Health Plan, patients, and the community?

Vision for the Future: Prism Health is a highly integrated health system in the Midwest that lives its public commitment of the Triple Aim. We provide high quality and safe patient care, and we are good stewards of our resources by providing cost-effective, affordable care, all while improving the health of our population. In providing these services, we strive to build a culture of collaboration between our health system facilities and our health plan to achieve the Triple Aim.

PART III

DEFINE

D1. **Situation & Scope**	D2. **Stakeholders, Difficulties, & Problem Areas**	D3. **Issue Statements & Problem Statement**
D1.1 Describe the *situation* D1.2 Scope the work	D2.1 Begin stakeholder analysis D2.2 Identify *difficulties* D2.3 Group difficulties into *problem areas*	D3.1 Create *issue statement* for each problem area D3.2 Create overall *problem statement* and vision for future

STUDY

S1. **Root Causes & Alternative Solutions**	S2. **Decision Criteria, Research, & Findings**	S3. **Conclusions**
S1.1 Generate possible root causes S1.2 Generate potential alternative solutions	S2.1 Develop decision criteria S2.2 Determine additional information needed S2.3 Develop *findings* through research S2.4 Review, reflect, and revise approach	S3.1 Collate, analyze, and judge the alternative solutions S3.2 Synthesize judgments into a set of *conclusions*

ACT

A1. **Recommendations & Milestones**	A2. **Communication Strategy & Consensus Building**	A3. **Implementation & Monitoring**
A1.1 Create integrated set of *recommendations* A1.2 Develop key implementation milestones	A2.1 Revisit stakeholder analysis A2.2 Create communication plan A2.3 Implement communication plan and validate approval/consensus of recommendations	A3.1 Develop detailed implementation plan A3.2 Monitor results against key performance indicators

PRACTICE THE STUDY PHASE

OVERVIEW OF PART III

Part III of the text provides the "how-to" practice chapters for the Study phase to help you learn each of the steps in this phase. There is one practice chapter per step (Chapters 9, 10, and 11), followed by the answer key for the practice activities in each of the Study phase chapters (Chapter 12). All of your work in the Study phase builds on your work in the Define phase, so Chapters 5 through 8 must be completed before you progress to Chapters 9 through 11.

The structure of each practice chapter is as follows:

- A brief overview of the step and its substeps
- The "how-to" of completing each substep
- Key steps to complete each substep
- Tips for completing each substep sucessfully
- Tools that support writing up your work in each substep

As you work your way through the "how-to" practice chapters, it will be very helpful for you to go back to Chapter 2 to read its corresponding detailed information regarding the "what" description for each Study phase substep.

Many of the activities use The Spinal Frontier case in Chapter 1 for you to practice the Problem Solving Method. The Chapter 12 Activity Key provides answers or suggested responses based on The Spinal Frontier case.

As you complete each chapter, you will complete a written product for each of the substeps in it. Thus, the practice chapters should be completed in order, because the work you complete in each practice chapter is used in the next one. Writing out your work is important for internalizing the method. As you gain experience in using the Problem-Solving Method, you will rarely write out the steps; they will instead be a part of your logical thought process.

Leave yourself time for uninterrupted attention to work through each chapter. The activities will require your thoughtful application.

CHAPTER 9

PRACTICE STUDY STEP S1: ROOT CAUSES AND ALTERNATIVE SOLUTIONS

OVERVIEW OF STUDY PHASE

Part III of the text covers the Study phase of the Problem-Solving Method, shown in Figure 9.1. The Study phase begins the second wave of divergent-convergent thinking of the Problem-Solving Method. It comprises three major steps, each of which has several substeps:

S1: Root Causes and Alternative Solutions (Chapter 9)

S2: Decision Criteria, Research and Findings (Chapter 10)

S3: Conclusions (Chapter 11)

As you move to the Study phase of the Problem-Solving Method, you build on what you have completed in the Define phase steps. In particular, you will be referring to your stakeholder analysis table and your problem area summary table.

The Study phase is conducted problem area by problem area. Based on the Chapter 8 Activity Key for the Define phase, four problem areas were identified: (a) Care Model; (b) Payer Relations; (c) Goal Misalignment; and (d) Decision-Making Process. So, you will be completing the Study phase steps for these four problem areas.

The structure of the Study phase practice chapters is identical to that of the Define phase. Each substep begins with a brief overview and a "how-to" description section, followed by the steps, tips, tools, and activities. As you work through these "how-to" practice chapters, remember to refer back to Chapter 2 for the indepth "what" description of each step and substep.

Chapter 12 contains the Activity Key example answers for the activities found in the three practice chapters for the Study phase.

When you have completed the Study phase, you will have developed conclusions about the relative merits of the alternative solutions for each problem area. These conclusions will, in turn, inform the final set of integrated recommendations in the Act phase.

STUDY

S1. Root Causes & Alternative Solutions	S2. Decision Criteria, Research, & Findings	S3. Conclusions
S1.1 Generate possible root causes S1.2 Generate potential alternative solutions	S2.1 Develop decision criteria S2.2 Determine additional information needed S2.3 Develop _findings_ through research S2.4 Review, reflect, and revise approach	S3.1 Collate, analyze, and judge the alternative solutions S3.2 Synthesize judgments into a set of _conclusions_

FIGURE 9.1 Study phase of the Problem-Solving Method.

STUDY STEP S1: ROOT CAUSES AND ALTERNATIVE SOLUTIONS

As shown in Figure 9.2, there are two substeps in the Root Causes and Alternative Solutions step in the Study phase of the Problem-Solving Method: S1.1, Generate possible root causes for each problem area; and S1.2, Generate potential alternative solutions.

Unlike the Define phase, where you had to stick to the facts when listing difficulties, in this first step of the Study phase, you are encouraged to brainstorm, speculate, and engage in divergent, creative thinking. For the difficulties in each problem area, you brainstorm a list of possible root causes. Then for each of the possible root causes, you brainstorm a list of potential alternative solutions that would eliminate or alleviate those root causes. At this point, you don't know the actual root causes or which alternative solutions are preferred. That is what you will research in Study phase step S2.

PRACTICE S1.1: GENERATE POSSIBLE ROOT CAUSES

Possible root causes are an extensive list of possible underlying reasons for the difficulties in a problem area.

HOW TO GENERATE POSSIBLE ROOT CAUSES

In this step, generate possible root causes that might be creating the set of difficulties in each problem area. In contrast to the issue statements and problem statement, which

STUDY

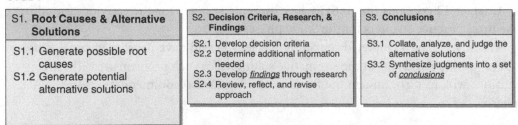

S1. Root Causes & Alternative Solutions	S2. Decision Criteria, Research, & Findings	S3. Conclusions
S1.1 Generate possible root causes S1.2 Generate potential alternative solutions	S2.1 Develop decision criteria S2.2 Determine additional information needed S2.3 Develop _findings_ through research S2.4 Review, reflect, and revise approach	S3.1 Collate, analyze, and judge the alternative solutions S3.2 Synthesize judgments into a set of _conclusions_

FIGURE 9.2 Study step S1: Root causes and alternative solutions.

require known facts, generating possible root causes encourages you to make some edu-cated guesses and hypothesize about why difficulties are occurring in each problem area. At this step, there is not yet enough information to ascertain the actual underlying root causes for the difficulties in the problem area. Some of your possible root causes may turn out to be actual root causes, while others will not. At this point, you just don't know.

You begin to identify possible root causes for each problem area by first reviewing the materials you have collected, summarized, and collated from the Define phase. The stakeholder analysis table provides perceived root causes that were provided to you by the stakeholders. You may have reviewed organizational data or reports that highlight other possible root causes. And, through directly observing processes, you may have noted possible root causes of process problems you observed. All of these sources help you brainstorm your initial list of possible root causes.

You need to expand beyond this initial list. There are a variety of ways to do this. Review published peer reviewed and trade journals. Talk to experts in the field. Use your professional network to identify others who may have faced a similar situation and talk with them. Interview additional stakeholders. These resources help identify additional possible root causes that should be considered.

In The Spinal Frontier case, for example, you may learn through reading and talking to experts that goal misalignment in a Triple Aim environment often occurs when employees are still evaluated based on productivity (i.e., number of surgeries or tests performed). But if the payment model is now outcome and value-based, more volume might not translate into more revenue for the organization. Thus, one possible root cause of the misaligned goals problem area could be that Prism is rewarding employees based on production volume or revenue production, not outcomes.

Brainstorming is also a productive way to generate ideas. As part of the brainstorm-ing process, utilizing Lean tools, such as asking the "5 Whys" and developing cause–effect (fishbone) diagrams, is also helpful. For each possible root cause generated, the "5 Whys" approach requires that you ask why that possible root cause is present. By asking this question iteratively "5 times" for each answer you come up with, it helps you delve deeper from what may be symptoms to ideas about what might be the underlying cause. Cause–effect diagrams facilitate a visual approach to identifying possible root causes for each difficulty in the problem area. Flowcharting a process can help identify where diffi-culties are occurring to generate ideas about possible root causes.

Remember to engage in divergent thinking when generating possible root causes. Do not judge and discard them at this stage. When you are done with this substep, you should have a list of possible root causes for the difficulties in each problem area.

Finally, in continuing with the "never assume" mindset, when problems arise in the organization in which you work, you must always consider the possibility that you are a possible root cause of a difficulty. As you review the problem areas and their difficulties, you should ask for feedback from others about ways in which your behavior, your work habits, your personality, your decision-making style, or other characteristics might be a possible root cause.

KEY STEPS TO GENERATE POSSIBLE ROOT CAUSES

Step 1: Review the possible root causes summarized in both your stakeholder analysis table from step D2.1 and the difficulties in the problem area summary table from step D3.1 of the Define phase.

Step 2: For each problem area, generate additional possible root causes for the difficulties. This can be done by brainstorming, additional discussions with stakeholders, interviewing persons who are experts in this area or may have faced a similar situation, reading published articles about the topic, contacting trade organizations or national best practice organizations, rounding, and direct observation.

Step 3: Add the additional possible root causes in the corresponding column of the problem area summary table from step D3.1 of the Define phase.

TIPS TO GENERATE POSSIBLE ROOT CAUSES

- There are a variety of tools and techniques from Lean methods and Design Thinking and Human-Centered Design that can facilitate brainstorming possible root causes. Learn and use these techniques.

- When rounding or directly observing to understand a process as part of identifying possible root causes, ensure you have the permission of the department and that all know why you are there. Be specific about what process you want to observe. Take very specific notes. Ask permission before taking pictures or recording. Set aside time with the leader or stakeholders in the area to debrief them on your observations and to further interview them to uncover root causes. Seek the input of those who engage in the process. The mindset of Lean when observing processes can be very helpful as you observe for possible root causes.

POSSIBLE ROOT CAUSES TOOL

As stated, any tools that support and structure creative idea generation are useful in this substep. Lean, Design Thinking, and Human-Centered Design all have tools to support idea generation.

The Problem-Solving Method tool that you use in this substep is the problem area summary table you created in step D3.1 of the Define phase. For each problem area, you update the "possible root causes" column to document your work in substep S1.1. Table 9.1 shows a problem area summary table that has been completed through the Define phase, using the Chapter 8 Activity Key answers for The Spinal Frontier. You would complete the last column of this table by adding your possible root causes for each problem area.

TABLE 9.1 Problem Area Summary Table for The Spinal Frontier Case

PROBLEM AREA	ISSUE STATEMENT	DIFFICULTIES*	POSSIBLE ROOT CAUSES
Care Model	What is the optimal care model for treating chronic neck and back pain, in light of the MedSpine joint venture proposal and resistance to it by some key stakeholders, Prism's high costs of providing spine care, the health plan's increasing focus on value-based care, and the health system's Triple Aim goal?	5, 7, 8, 9, 10, 12, 14, 15	
Payer Relations	How can Prism Health System best leverage the expertise and resources of its health plan to achieve the Triple Aim, given that the health plan's CEO has expressed concerns about the health system's ability to provide value-based care?	7,8	
Goal Misalign-ment	How can Prism Health System align the goals of its Musculoskeletal Clin-ical Service Line to its commitment to the Triple Aim, in light of Prism's high costs of spine care compared to insurance industry benchmarks, and the Service Line's reliance on volume, activity, and revenue data to judge the success of the service line?	5, 11, 13	
Decision-Making Process	What is the appropriate deci-sion-making process for the Musculo-skeletal Clinical Service Line, in light of the current composition, leader-ship, operating, and authority struc-ture of its Steering Committee, and the concerns expressed by several key stakeholders on the Committee that they have not had input into the MedSpine joint venture?	1, 2, 3, 4, 6, 9, 15	

*See numbered list of difficulties in Chapter 8, Activity 14.

Problem Statement: What is the optimal care model for patients with chronic neck and back pain that aligns with Prism Health System's Triple Aim goal, in light of the MedSpine joint venture proposal, the high costs of Prism's spine care, and the health plan's focus on value-based care; and what are the implications of the care model for payer relations and the decision-making structure of the service line—to the satisfaction of the Service Line Steering Committee, the Prism Health Plan, patients, and the community?

Vision for the Future: Prism Health is a highly integrated health system in the Midwest that lives its public commitment of the Triple Aim. We provide high quality and safe patient care, and we are good stewards of our resources by providing cost-effective, affordable care, all while improving the health of our population. In providing these services, we strive to build a culture of collaboration between our health system facilities and our health plan to achieve the Triple Aim.

ACTIVITIES TO GENERATE POSSIBLE ROOT CAUSES

You will continue to use The Spinal Frontier case for the activities, building on your work in the Define phase that you completed in Chapters 5, 6, and 7.

■ STUDY ACTIVITY 1

Generate possible root causes for the difficulties you have listed in the problem area summary table, and add them to the last column in the table. Remember to focus on one problem area at a time when generating possible root causes.

■ STUDY ACTIVITY 2

Find a resource that describes how to create a cause-effect (fishbone) diagram. Create a cause-effect diagram for each of the problem areas in The Spinal Frontier.

PRACTICE S1.2: GENERATE POTENTIAL ALTERNATIVE SOLUTIONS

Potential alternative solutions are an extensive list of actions that might make the possible root causes listed in Study phase step S1.1 disappear if implemented.

GENERATE POTENTIAL ALTERNATIVE SOLUTIONS

Alternative solutions are different possible answers to the "how" part of the question posed in the issue statement of each problem area. Each possible root cause you generated in the Study step S1.1 requires at least one potential alternative solution that, if implemented, would eliminate that possible root cause. The potential alternative solutions must be action-oriented, although "do nothing" (status quo) is always an alternative. "Do more research" is *not* an action-oriented alternative. Potential alternative solutions do not need to be mutually exclusive.

KEY STEPS TO GENERATE POTENTIAL ALTERNATIVE SOLUTIONS

Step 1: Review the suggested alternative solutions from your stakeholder interviews summarized in your stakeholder analysis table from Define step D2.1 as a starting point for potential alternative solutions.

Step 2: Be resourceful in tapping a vast array of resources to brainstorm additional alternatives—continued discussion with stakeholders, published literature on the topic, web sites, industry contacts, subject matter experts, and your professional network.

Step 3: Document the alternative solutions within each problem area by adding a new column called "potential alternative solutions" to the problem area summary table. Map the alternative solutions to the root causes within each problem area.

TIPS TO GENERATE POTENTIAL ALTERNATIVE SOLUTIONS

- Do not rule out any alternatives at this phase. Have the imagination, creativity, and courage to arrive at novel, innovative alternatives. Do not assume at the outset that the wildest alternative cannot be implemented, and do not worry at this step as to what is the "best" or "best acceptable" alternative solution, or whether any alternative is "right" or "wrong."

- The alternatives should be action oriented, not process oriented. Except in extreme circumstances, a solution of forming a committee to further study the problem or hiring a consultant are process solutions that should be avoided.

- Ask yourself the following questions when brainstorming potential alternative solutions:

  o What alternative solutions could eliminate, reduce or avoid the possible root causes and the difficulties identified?

  o What are creative, innovative alternatives to attain "what ought to be"?

  o What alternative solutions are preferred by the stakeholders?

  o What alternative solutions are generated via observing the current situation/process and debriefing with stakeholders?

  o What are the benchmark/best practice alternative solutions?

  o What alternatives could be considered in the short-term versus long-term?

  o What alternative solutions have been tested in other organizations or are noted in literature and research?

- Ask yourself the following questions when reviewing the set of potential alternative solutions you have generated:

  o Do the potential alternative solutions creatively stretch the limits of what might be "possible" rather than just including only those that are "feasible"?

  o Have alternative solutions been established for each of the problem areas in the problem statement?

  o Are the alternative solutions imaginative and comprehensive?

  o Do the alternatives include those preferred by those with final decision-making authority? By those who may significantly influence the decision? By those who will be responsible for implementing the final set of recommended alternatives? By those who will be affected by the organizational changes resulting from the recommended alternatives?

    o   Do the alternative solutions provide substantive action-oriented solutions to the significant difficulties? Are they potential action-oriented answers to the "how" question in the problem area's issue statement?

■   If you find yourself creating the same set of potential alternative solutions across at least two problem areas, it may indicate that there is enough overlap between your problem areas that you may want to revisit whether you should revise how you have grouped your difficulties.

POTENTIAL ALTERNATIVE SOLUTIONS TOOL

Brainstorming is the main tool used to generate potential alternative solutions. Talking to experts and colleagues and reading literature will also help you identify potential alternative solutions. Similar to generating possible root causes, generating potential alternative solutions is also completed one problem area at a time.

When you are done, add a column called "potential alternative solutions" to the problem area summary table, as shown in Table 9.2.

ACTIVITIES TO GENERATE POTENTIAL ALTERNATIVE SOLUTIONS

■ STUDY ACTIVITY 3

List the preferred alternative solutions from your stakeholder analysis table for The Spinal Frontier case into the appropriate row corresponding to its problem area in the problem area summary table (Table 9.2).

■ STUDY ACTIVITY 4

Generate additional potential alternative solutions. Ask yourself the questions in the tips section when generating them. Generate at least one potential alternative solution in each problem area by reading published literature on the topic, and at least one of them by speaking to an industry contact or a subject matter expert.

TABLE 9.2 Problem Area Summary Table With Potential Alternative Solutions Column

PROBLEM AREA	ISSUE STATEMENT	DIFFICULTIES	POSSIBLE ROOT CAUSES	POTENTIAL ALTERNATIVE SOLUTIONS
Care Model				
Payer Relations				
Goal Misalignment				
Decision-Making Process				

■ STUDY ACTIVITY 5

Add your potential alternative solutions to the problem area summary table. Check to make sure each possible root cause has at least one potential alternative solution. Review your generated set of potential alternative solutions for each problem area, and ask yourself the questions in the tips section when reviewing them.

CHAPTER 10

PRACTICE STUDY STEP S2: DECISION CRITERIA, RESEARCH, AND FINDINGS

STUDY STEP S2: DECISION CRITERIA, RESEARCH, AND FINDINGS

As shown in Figure 10.1, there are four substeps in the Decision Criteria, Research, and Findings step in the Study phase of the Problem-Solving Method: S2.1, Develop decision criteria; S2.2, Determine additional information needed; S2.3, Develop findings through research; and S2.4, Review, reflect, and revise approach.

Remember to go back to Chapter 2 to read the "what" of Step S2 before starting the practice of the "how" in this chapter.

One of the most important things to remember as you complete this step is that as you research the merits of the potential alternative solutions, you need to pay attention to all of the evidence. You do not want to fall into the trap of confirmation bias, where you only pay attention to findings that support your point of view. You need to remain impartial as you conduct your research, and not insert your judgment or preferences into your findings. You can report others' judgments or preferences, identifying whose they are, in your findings, but you can't include your own. You refrain from injecting your judgment about your findings during this step.

It is also important during this step to keep the stakeholders and their viewpoints at the top of your mind. Referring to the stakeholder analysis during this phase will be important. If your findings appear to indicate that a solution preferred by a key stakeholder is not likely going to be a candidate for recommendation, you need to develop a plan for circling back with the stakeholder to discuss what you are finding.

PRACTICE S2.1: DEVELOP DECISION CRITERIA

Decision criteria are the factors that will be used to judge the relative merits of the potential alternative solutions.

HOW TO DEVELOP DECISION CRITERIA

You need well-defined decision criteria to evaluate the strengths and weaknesses and pros and cons of the potential alternative solutions that you have generated for each

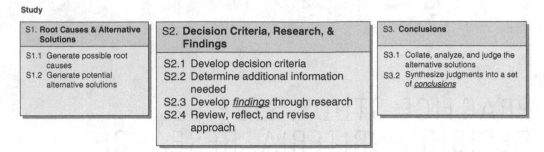

FIGURE 10.1 Study step S2: Decision criteria, research, and findings.

problem area. To develop decision criteria, look at your stakeholder analysis and issue statement to see if it helps identify any that are specific to this situation. Then, determine if there are general decision criteria that are particularly salient for judging the set of alternatives, such as budget or cost, implementation time frame, and acceptability to various key stakeholder groups.

At this substep of the process, you do not have the information required to identify the best acceptable alternative solutions, as you have not yet conducted any research to identify actual root causes and determine the relative merits of the alternatives you have generated based on your decision criteria.

KEY STEPS TO DEVELOP DECISION CRITERIA

Step 1: Go back to your stakeholder analysis, your issue statements, and your vision for the future to review their goals. Determine what decision criteria could be used based on those goals. See the tips that follow for examples of additional decision criteria that are relevant in many situations.

Step 2: Create a definition for each criteria. In this definition, if possible, articulate a measured goal that indicates how you will judge if you met the established criteria. For instance, goals could be to increase patient satisfaction scores by 10%, increase provider engagement scores by 10%, generate 5% cost savings, achieve a 2% incremental increase in the operating margin, all of which can be achieved within one year.

Step 3: Create a problem area decision criteria table that you will use to summarize your findings once you have conducted research to evaluate your alternative solutions relative to the decision criteria. You will begin to populate the cells of the table as you conduct your research in Study substep 2.3, and will complete it in Study substep 3.1.

TIPS TO DEVELOP DECISION CRITERIA

■   Do not make any judgments in this step about the merits of your potential alternative solutions. This will come later in the process.

- Healthcare-specific criteria in common use today include the Institute for Healthcare Improvement's Triple Aim, which has been expanded to the Quadruple Aim.

  o *Patient Experience:* How does the alternative solution improve the patient experience in terms of quality of care, outcomes, and patient satisfaction?

  o *Cost of Care/Efficiency:* What are the costs of care for this alternative? Does this alternative reduce the per capita cost of care at the community level?

  o *Population Health/Community:* Does this alternative improve health at the population or community level?

  o *Provider Engagement and Satisfaction:* How does this alternative enhance employees' and other providers' experience of providing care and services to patients?

- Other typical decision criteria may include:

  o *Time:* Is the time frame this solution takes to be implemented acceptable given the problem? If a short-term solution is needed within a week, an alternative that takes 2 months to implement will not be acceptable. In these situations, you may need a short-term solution to "stop the hemorrhage" and a longer-term solution to eliminate the root cause of the hemorrhage.

  o *Cost/Budget:* How much does this alternative cost to implement and maintain? Is it within budget? Is that cost justifiable given its likely benefit? Some alternatives may be more costly, but provide greater benefit to the organization. Does the alternative meet a financial threshold specified by the organization? Most investment decisions undergo financial analysis to determine their cash flow and rate of return, for example.

  o *Organizational Culture and Mission, Vision, and Values:* Does the alternative solution fit the organization's culture? Its mission, vision, and values?

  o *Broader Environmental Context:* How well does this alternative respond to the local, state, or national political and social climates? To market pressures? To local community expectations or standards?

  o *Legal:* Are there legislative policies underway that might change rules or regulations at the state or federal level that would impact the alternatives? Is there any pending or current litigation inside or outside your organization that has implications for the alternatives?

  o *Compliance:* Does this alternative violate any internal compliance policies or procedures? Would it require the organization to create new policies or procedures? What is your organization's compliance department's view about the relative merits of the alternatives with respect to compliance?

  o *Ethical:* Are there any personal, professional, organizational, community, or societal ethical dilemmas that arise from this alternative solution? Is there conflict between stakeholder groups that this solution exacerbates? If so, what will it take to overcome them?

o   *Innovation:* Is this solution creative? Does it step outside the realm of current approaches to solve the problem?

o   *Stakeholder Views:* What were the various stakeholders' views about this alternative, both pro and con? What would it take for unfavorable views of this alternative to be overcome?

DECISION CRITERIA TOOL

After you have identified the decision criteria that are relevant to use for the problem area, you should create a problem area decision criteria table. As shown in Table 10.1, the alternative solutions are listed one per row, and each column is a decision criteria and its definition. The table will remain blank until you have completed your research and additional interviews in S2.3. An example problem area decision criteria table follows. Each problem area requires its own table.

ACTIVITIES TO DEVELOP DECISION CRITERIA

Review the alternative solutions you have developed for each problem area of The Spinal Frontier case.

■ STUDY ACTIVITY 6

Develop the decision criteria against which your alternative solutions in each problem area should be judged.

■ STUDY ACTIVITY 7

Create a problem area decision criteria table for each of your problem areas in The Spinal Frontier case.

TABLE 10.1 Problem Area Decision Criteria Table

PROBLEM AREA NAME	CRITERIA 1	CRITERIA 2	CRITERIA 3	CRITERIA 4
	Criteria 1 Definition	Criteria 2 Definition	Criteria 3 Definition	Criteria 4 Definition
Alternative Solution 1				
Alternative Solution 2				
More alternatives to follow				

PRACTICE S2.2: DETERMINE ADDITIONAL INFORMATION NEEDED

Additional information needed is what you need to know to determine the strengths and weaknesses and pros and cons of your potential alternative solutions relative to your decision criteria, and whether a potential root cause is an actual root cause.

HOW TO DETERMINE ADDITIONAL INFORMATION NEEDED

Given your decision criteria, you need to conduct research to determine how each of the alternative solutions compares against the criteria. What information will you need, given your decision criteria? In addition, the hypothesized root causes need to be investigated to identify actual root causes. Write the information needed in the form of research questions. For example, if "time needed for implementation" is a criteria, "In what time frame can alternative X be implemented?" would be an example of a research question. Based on the information needed, you develop a research plan to gather the information.

Often, a subset of the information you need is from organizational data systems. This will typically require that you submit a special request for a data pull or a data report. You will need to be able to articulate what data you need, and study the organization's data dictionaries to get an understanding of what data elements being captured by the organization correspond to the data you need. You will likely need to meet with the organizational data analyst who is knowledgeable about the data to ensure you are getting the appropriate data, and whether they can run the analytics to answer the questions to which you need answers, or whether they will pull data and expect that you can run the analysis.

This can be a time-consuming process, with long delay times from the time you request the data to the time you receive it. Data requests should be submitted as early as possible to ensure you receive the data set in the time frame required and have sufficient time to analyze it as part of your research process needed to study the problem.

KEY STEPS TO DETERMINE ADDITIONAL INFORMATION NEEDED

Step 1: Review each problem area decision criteria table and determine what you need to know in order to complete its cells. Also, for the potential root causes for which those alternatives have been generated, what do you need to know to determine if it is an actual root cause?

Step 2: Based on the information you need, develop research questions that, when answered, would provide you with that information.

Step 3: For each research question, determine what source you will use to find the answer. Examples could include reading published literature, conducting surveys, requesting and analyzing organizational data, interviewing experts and industry contacts, talking to stakeholders, observing and mapping core processes, pilot testing an alternative, and so on.

Step 4: Collate your information needs by source to create one consolidated research plan that spans all of your problem areas. This research plan helps you organize what questions you will ask or study from each of the sources.

TIPS TO DETERMINE ADDITIONAL INFORMATION NEEDED

- You may discover that additional decision criteria are needed during this step. If this is the case, add the criteria and definition/measure to the table, and develop any additional research questions that arise.

- Share your decision criteria tables and your research plan with your organizational preceptor. They may have additional insights to build on what you developed thus far, and may be able to provide you with useful contacts or sources for your research plan.

- If you are a student project team, or if you are relatively new in your tenure in the organization, you should review your research plan with the person to whom you are accountable for the project. They will often have advice about people in the organization or community who could best answer some of the questions you need answered when you do your research. They will also have insights about the power structure and culture of the organization, as well as social, economic, and political aspects that may be relevant to the problem, but of which you are unaware. When in doubt, ask for input.

- As you identify the information needed to develop a research plan, the following questions are often useful to ask yourself:

  o What external and internal data do you already have related to the alternatives? What additional data will you need? Do you know what questions you are seeking to answer through data requests? Do you have a clear data request underway?

  o Have you observed the process(es) that may be associated with the problem?

  o Do you understand the context—what is the history, culture, climate, and environment of this organization? This is particularly difficult to discern as a student or new graduate, and you will need to make sure you talk with your organizational preceptors, mentors and other experienced leaders to get experiential knowledge about the unique challenges different contexts or cultures might create in choosing among alternatives.

  o What has been historically important in the organization; for example, political, cultural, financial, public, ethical legal, demographic and marketplace considerations, time factors, special needs of stakeholders?

o   What "type" of case are you facing to aid you in identifying areas of consideration? Is this primarily a case about mergers, joint ventures, human resource issues, union issues, operational throughput, business development, reorganization? Have you sought subject matter expertise on the topic to learn more about the common issues for this type of problem and how they might affect the merits of different alternative solutions?

o   Have you reviewed your stakeholder analysis to determine if you have considered all the relevant stakeholders? Do you need more information from those you have already interviewed?

ADDITIONAL INFORMATION NEEDED TOOL

All of the questions you generate in totality represent the areas of research you need to conduct to gather information to answer those questions. You will need to organize these questions into a research plan. An example plan is shown in Table 10.2. It summarizes the information needed, the source of the information, data or questions the information needs to answer, the date the data or information are needed, and the status of the data gathering activities. Update the status column as you gather information to keep track of where you are in the research process. Also, revise your interview guide from Define substep D2.1 as needed (see Exhibit 6.1).

ACTIVITY TO DETERMINE ADDITIONAL INFORMATION NEEDED

■ STUDY ACTIVITY 8

For each problem area, generate the information needed in the form of research questions.

■ STUDY ACTIVITY 9

Develop a research plan in a similar format to that shown in the research plan tool.

PRACTICE S2.3: DEVELOP FINDINGS THROUGH RESEARCH

Findings are the objective, factual answers you learn through conducting your research.

HOW TO DEVELOP FINDINGS THROUGH RESEARCH

Findings are statements of fact, people's opinions, or values that are stated as such (along with their underlying rationale for that opinion), and data analysis results. Findings offer evidence about the actual root causes of the difficulties and the evidence for or against the alternative solutions in each problem area.

TABLE 10.2 Research Plan for Information Needed

PROJECT RESEARCH PLAN

Organization

Team Members

NUMBER	INFORMATION NEEDED	SOURCE OF INFORMATION	QUESTIONS/DATA REQUEST	DATE NEEDED BY	STATUS
1	Current costs for spine patients	Finance	Costs by provider, costs by surgery, note inpatient and outpatient. Include DRGs and procedure codes	2 weeks	Need to submit data request through CFO in order to expedite the request
2	Cost benchmarks used by the Prism Health Plan	Prism analytics	What benchmarks does Prism Health Plan use and can the group have access?	2 weeks	Work with Prism CFO and Health Plan CFO to determine how to access
3	Spine Center of Excellence Best Practices	National consulting firms, professional societies focused on spine care, literature review, interviews with analogous organizations with spine centers	What are the best practices in organizing spine care in a large delivery system?	3 weeks	Team to split up sources and bring back research to team meeting in 3 weeks. Shared document created to add findings.
4					
5					

The process of developing your findings, based on your research plan, is called your research. You must include all relevant findings, not simply those that support your preferred alternative solution or negate alternatives you do not favor. As such, this research step is analytical, and focuses on facts. *Findings must exclude your personal judgments and values.*

KEY STEPS TO DEVELOP FINDINGS THROUGH RESEARCH

Step 1: Use your research plan to complete your research. Your research should include interviewing stakeholders and industry experts, analyzing data, reviewing organizational reports, observing processes and meetings, and reading relevant literature and industry websites.

Step 2: Summarize and document all findings, and place the relevant findings into the appropriate cell of the decision table.

TIPS TO DEVELOP FINDINGS THROUGH RESEARCH

- Data requests and scheduling interviews sometimes require long lead times to get them fulfilled. Try to get data requests in as soon as possible and get on key stakeholders' calendars as soon as you know you want to talk with them. Your organizational preceptor may need to do what they can to facilitate your data pull request getting fulfilled by the organization.

- Your program's alumni are often good sources to contact when conducting your research. They may be able to answer your questions and to connect you to others in their organization with whom you could speak who could answer your questions.

- In the course of conducting your research, it is common to learn of new potential alternative solutions. Add them to your problem area summary table tool and your decision criteria table, and generate any new information needed to add questions to your research plan to address the new alternative.

- Soon after each interview or literature review, summarize your findings from your interview notes while they are still fresh in your mind.

- When completing the decision criteria table with your findings, you can either summarize them directly in the table, or you can create a master list of numbered findings, and then include only the numbers in the appropriate cells of the table. You can also use a sticky note exercise in this step.

- Some of your industry experts might say to do "X" alternative. If they do, you need to probe to understand the underlying rationale for why they recommend that alternative rather than the others. Probe for the pros and cons, the strengths and weaknesses. Otherwise, the finding will simply be that "Expert A says to do X," which is not helpful to you.

- In doing your research, you may rule out some potential root causes as not being true. If this is the case, then any alternatives that were in the set solely to eliminate that root cause should no longer be in consideration, since they will fix nothing.

- Remember that the findings must exclude your personal judgments and values. To exclude relevant findings because they do not support your biases or points of view is unethical. It is important that you maintain objectivity, as if you are an external consultant stepping outside of yourself and your personal preferences and biases, as you review and reflect on all you are discovering through your research.

- As you conduct research, you may uncover new difficulties and problem areas. To avoid scope creep, talk with your preceptor, boss, or team to determine whether the scope needs to be revised, and if it is to be expanded, the implications for the timeline, budget, and resources for solving the problem. Or, if a new problem area needs to be included, are there other problem areas that should be excluded?

RESEARCH FINDINGS TOOL

As you conduct research, it can be very easy to lose sight of where you are and what you are learning. As you complete gathering information from each source, you should take the time soon after completing the interview, reading, or data analysis to summarize what you have learned about each alternative relative to the decision criteria. The problem area decision criteria table (Table 10.3) is where you should summarize your findings in one location. An example is shown in Table 10.3.

Depending on the volume of findings you produce through your research, it may not be feasible to create an easy-to-read table. Instead, you can create a numbered list of your findings and use the numbers, rather than the text itself, in the appropriate cell of the table.

ACTIVITIES TO DEVELOP FINDINGS THROUGH RESEARCH

■ STUDY ACTIVITY 10

Review the research plan you developed in Study step S2.2, and split up the workload among three or four classmates. Each of you should gain practice in conducting at

TABLE 10.3 Populating the Problem Area Decision Criteria Table

PROBLEM AREA 1	CRITERIA 1	CRITERIA 2	CRITERIA 3	CRITERIA 4
	Criteria 1 Definition	Criteria 2 Definition	Criteria 3 Definition	Criteria 4 Definition
Alternative Solution 1	Finding # 1,5, 7		Finding # 2,6	
Alternative Solution 2, etc.				

least one interview and reviewing at least one published article or industry website as part of your research.

■ STUDY ACTIVITY 11

Create a numbered master list of all of your findings. Using a whiteboard with your decision criteria table drawn on it, write finding numbers on sticky notes and place them in the appropriate cells of the decision table. Microsoft Excel or Google Sheets can facilitate this activity. For each cell, write a summary of the findings. The summary should not include your judgment or opinions.

PRACTICE S2.4: REVIEW, REFLECT, AND REVISE APPROACH

Review, reflect, and revise are a "hard stop" for you to review all the work that you have conducted in all of the steps so far.

HOW TO REVIEW, REFLECT, AND REVISE APPROACH

This is the time to take a step back and review the landscape of all the work you have completed so far. Especially during the research phase, you may uncover new stakeholders, new difficulties, new problem areas, new possible root causes, and/or new potential alternative solutions. If you have, you need to circle back to earlier steps to update and revise them. You should meet with one or more key stakeholder groups to update them on your work to date and what you have found to get their feedback and insights.

KEY STEPS TO REVIEW, REFLECT, AND REVISE APPROACH

Step 1: Ensure all of your relevant findings are accurately summarized in the decision criteria table.

Step 2: Review all of your work so far, paying particular attention to your findings and whether any of them indicate the need to revise or update any work in your previous steps.

Step 3: Review your stakeholder analysis, problem areas, issue statements, and difficulties to determine if the logic trail is evident from problem areas to potential alternative solutions. Revise if necessary.

Step 4: Schedule a meeting with your preceptors to discuss your work to date. Incorporate their feedback into your work. Discuss if any changes need to be made to the scope of work for the project based on what you have found.

Step 5: Review your stakeholder analysis table and your findings in your decision criteria table to see if there are alternatives preferred by one or more stakeholder groups for which the findings do not look favorable. Talk to your organizational precep-tor about how to best connect with these stakeholder groups to update them on what you have found so far.

TIPS TO REVIEW, REFLECT, AND REVISE APPROACH

- When meeting with stakeholders to review your work, avoid using prob-lem-solving "lingo" from the Problem-Solving Method (e.g., using words like difficulties, issue statements, and problem statement). Talk in lay language that makes logical sense to those who have not been exposed to the Method.

- Avoid sharing all of the excruciating details of each of your steps during the stakeholder meetings. Summarize your work and focus on the key points, putting all of this in a written format they can take with them to review later if they wish. Include your contact information on the documents in case they want to contact you later with additional feedback.

- Bring your signed consulting agreement with you to the meeting with your organizational preceptor. If your work to date indicates the need to revise your scope of work, remember to update the consulting agreement, with all parties signing it again to ensure all are aware of the changes and it is documented. Beware of "scope creep" where more work gets added to the scope. If some-thing gets added to the scope within the same time frame for completion, then generally something else should be removed from the scope if no additional resources are provided.

TOOLS TO REVIEW, REFLECT, AND REVISE APPROACH

The relevant tools for this step are to review the completed tables you have completed so far. Review them to assess what you have learned.

For example, go back and review your problem area summary table that summarized your problem areas, issue statement, possible root causes and potential alternative solu-tions, problem statement, and vision for the future. With that in mind, next review your problem area decision criteria table. Are your findings providing you with information that will help you answer the questions posed in your issue statements? Are there any holes in your findings that suggest you need to conduct some additional research?

In addition, review your stakeholder analysis table. Given your findings, do some alternatives appear to be rising to the top for recommendation? How might different stakeholders respond to the facts and their implication for the various alternative solu-tions? How might you address potential opposition by stakeholders now before you get further into drawing conclusions and making recommendations?

APPLICATION TO REVIEW, REFLECT, AND REVISE APPROACH

■ STUDY ACTIVITY 12

Put together a written summary of your work so far on The Spinal Frontier case that you would share with the Prism Health System organizational preceptors.

■ STUDY ACTIVITY 13

Role play how you would share your progress to date during a mock meeting with the Prism Health System organizational preceptors.

CHAPTER 11

PRACTICE STUDY STEP S3: CONCLUSIONS

STUDY STEP S3: CONCLUSIONS

As shown in Figure 11.1, there are two substeps in the Conclusions step in the Study phase of the Problem Solving Method: S3.1, Collate, analyze, and judge the alternative solutions; and S3.2, Synthesize judgments into a set of conclusions.

Remember to go back to Chapter 2 to read the "what" of Study step S3 before starting the practice of the "how" in this chapter.

Recall that in Study substep S2.3, Develop findings through research, you were required to stick to the facts in your findings. Your findings can include other people's judgments about the relative merits of your alternative solutions, indicating in your findings whose judgments they are. But the findings cannot include your judgments or conclusions.

It is in Study step S3 that your judgment and conclusions come to the forefront. The logic of how you arrived at your judgment and conclusions should be clear to anyone who reviews your work.

PRACTICE S3.1: COLLATE, ANALYZE, AND JUDGE THE ALTERNATIVE SOLUTIONS

Collate, analyze, and judge the alternative solutions is the process of organizing and summarizing your findings relative to your decision criteria, and applying your judgment to what the findings are telling you about the merits of the alternative solutions.

HOW TO COLLATE, ANALYZE, AND JUDGE THE ALTERNATIVE SOLUTIONS

Review all of the notes you have taken as you conducted your research. Make sure you have organized and summarized all of the relevant findings into a numbered list. Complete the process of collating your findings into the appropriate cells in the problem area decision criteria table.

Next, review your completed problem area decision criteria table. It should have all of your findings summarized in the appropriate cells of the table.

Study

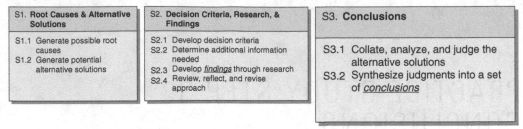

FIGURE 11.1 Study step S3: Conclusions.

Read through each row of the table (remember, each row lists one alternative). Based on your findings, what are *your* judgments about each alternative solution? What do *you* think are the pros and cons, and strengths and weaknesses, and why? Your logic should be clear, and you should be able to succinctly justify your answers clearly to anyone who would ask you for your rationale based on the facts you have collated.

As you review the findings for each alternative it may be helpful to apply formal decision support tools to the judgment process. A couple of examples are force field analysis[1] and decision analysis.[2] Force field analysis is a tool in which you identify the driving forces (the pros) and the restraining forces (the cons) acting on the alternative. You then assign a numerical score (e.g., 1 = weak through 5 = strong) to each of the driving and restraining forces and then sum the scores to see whether the scores are higher for the driving or restraining forces. Done with a team, the scoring process helps to clarify through discussion the strength of the forces for and against each alternative.

Decision analysis is an approach that assigns numerical scales to preferences. In this approach each of the decision criteria receives a numerical weight. Each of the levels of how well the alternative does on each decision criteria is assigned a score based on the level achieved. The final score for each alternative is calculated by multiplying the numerical weight of each decision criteria by the score of the level achieved on that criteria, and then summing across the decision criteria to arrive at a final score for each alternative under consideration.

Approaches that assign numerical scores to help you rank the alternatives can be helpful because rarely will one alternative dominate across all of the decision criteria. Some alternatives will be better on some decision criteria, while other alternatives will be superior on others. The discipline of developing scoring methods can help clarify your thinking.

This does not mean that you should always develop numerical scores before making judgments. Numerical scores can be helpful in certain situations; for example, for decisions that have large financial implications for the organization, when there is a high level of risk involved in the decision, or when there is disagreement among your team members about your judgments of the relative merits of the alternatives.

To summarize your judgments into one location, you should write out a numbered list that articulates your assessment of the pros and cons, and strengths and weaknesses of each alternative. Then, add a column at the far right called "judgments" in the problem area decision criteria table. In that column, complete each cell by typing in the numbers corresponding to the numbers of the relevant judgments that apply to that cell.

There are now three documents that you should review to trace your logic from your findings to your conclusions: (a) your numbered list of findings; (b) your numbered list of judgments; and (c) your completed problem area decision criteria table. For each alternative solution, read through the findings and judgments you have recorded as relevant for that alternative. Does the logic for each alternative's judgments logically flow from your findings? Are your judgments for each alternative sound and convincing?

Is there disagreement among the team as to the judgments of the alternative, even when working off of the same set of facts? If so, you need to figure out as a team what is driving that disagreement. Is it that different team members are weighting the decision criteria differently? If so, how might you resolve those differences? (Think about who your ultimate customer is—perhaps they should be the ones weighting the decision criteria.)

This substep is a difficult one because it requires higher-order thinking skills. That is, you are having to synthesize and integrate information across a variety of sources to arrive at your judgments about the alternatives.

KEY STEPS TO COLLATE, ANALYZE, AND JUDGE THE ALTERNATIVE SOLUTIONS

Step 1: Review your findings one last time to ensure that all of the relevant information from your research notes is captured, and that all relevant findings are collated in your decision criteria table. You should have collated information along the way in the Study phase, although this is the last time you are checking your research results—so make sure all findings are collated.

Step 2: Analyze the findings against the criteria and create a summary judgment for each alternative. What are the pros and cons, and the strengths and weaknesses of each alternative relative to the criteria?

Step 3: Add a column called "judgment" into each of your problem area decision criteria tables. Summarize your statements of judgment about each alternative into the decision criteria table.

Step 4: For each of your alternatives, review your findings and judgments used for that alternative to ensure that your logic is clear and convincing.

TIPS TO COLLATE, ANALYZE, AND JUDGE THE ALTERNATIVE SOLUTIONS

- Creating numbered lists of judgments can facilitate completing the problem area decision criteria table using the respective numbers in the judgment column, rather than the actual written text of the judgments.

- Comparisons of alternatives can often be facilitated by assigning numerical judgments to how well the alternatives fulfill the criteria. Examples include force field analysis,[1] and decision analysis.[2]

TOOL TO COLLATE, ANALYZE, AND JUDGE THE ALTERNATIVE SOLUTIONS

As described, tools that provide guidance for how to assign numerical scores to decision criteria and your findings can facilitate your ability to develop your judgments about the alternatives. Force field analysis and decision analysis are two examples of tools that were mentioned previously.

The tool used to document your judgments is the problem area decision criteria table. You add a column called "Your Judgments" that you populate with the numbers of the judgments in your numbered judgment list that are relevant for that alternative solution. See Table 11.1 for an example.

ACTIVITIES TO COLLATE, ANALYZE, AND JUDGE THE ALTERNATIVE SOLUTIONS

■ STUDY ACTIVITY 14

For each problem area in The Spinal Frontier, review the alternatives relative to your findings for each criteria. Based on your analysis, summarize the pros and cons, and strengths and weaknesses of the alternatives as a numbered list. Enter the numbers into the judgment column of the decision criteria table, indicating which are pro for the alternative and which are con.

PRACTICE S3.2: SYNTHESIZE JUDGMENTS INTO A SET OF CONCLUSIONS

Conclusions are statements that synthesize your judgments about the relative merits of the potential alternatives, and which are preferred or not, based on your distillation, synthesis, and interpretation of the findings.

HOW TO SYNTHESIZE JUDGMENTS INTO A SET OF CONCLUSIONS

In this substep, review your judgments for each of your alternatives, looking back to also review the findings that led to those judgments. As you look across all of your alternatives and your judgments about them, which alternatives rise to the top as contenders, and which do not? Why?

As you write conclusions, they are not simply regurgitations of your judgments. Instead, you are integrating and synthesizing your judgments into a smaller set of statements that summarize the merits of each alternative, and how the alternatives that you view as the main contenders compare to each other.

Novices to the Problem-Solving Method often write conclusions as action-oriented recommendations. For example, *"Enter into a joint venture with MedSpine"* is

TABLE 11.1 Judgment Column Added to Problem Area Decision Criteria Table*

CARE MODEL	PATIENT OUTCOMES	PATIENT SATISFACTION	CLINICIAN ACCEPTANCE	TOTAL COST OF CARE	HEALTH SYSTEM OPERATING MARGIN	TIMEFRAME TO IMPLEMENT	COST TO IMPLEMENT	YOUR JUDGMENTS
Criteria Measure	↑ by x%	↑ by x%	↑ by x%	↓ by x%	↑ by x%	< x months	< $ Cost	
Do Nothing- Status Quo				# 1,4				
Joint Venture	#2, 3a, 3b	#3a,b	#3d, 3e	#3f, 3g	#1, 3f, 3g, 4			
Alternative Solution 3...								

*The numbers in the cells correspond to the numbered findings in the example answers in the Study Activity 11 Key in Chapter 12.

an action-oriented recommendation, it is not a conclusion. As written, this statement provides no information about the logic of why a MedSpine joint venture is the preferred course of action. If your judgments lead you to conclude that a joint venture with MedSpine is a preferred option, and assuming you had judgments for the status quo alternative that are mostly cons or weaknesses, your conclusions might read as follows:

The MedSpine joint venture option is well aligned with the changing reimbursement models that drive value over volume, and Prism Health System's commitment to the cost, quality, and access goals of the Triple Aim. MedSpine's published clinical trials have documented cost-effective care with superior patient outcomes and high patient satisfaction with their nonsurgical approaches to treating chronic neck and back pain.

Maintaining Prism Health System's current care model that focuses on surgery and imaging for chronic neck and back pain is not sustainable. Our competitors are providing new nonsurgical treatments, and our own health plan may not choose us as a partner for their Spine Center of Distinction because our costs are high relative to their benchmarks.

As you read the conclusions, you can see that they provide a logic trail from the findings you developed through your research in Study phase substep S2.3, and the judgments you reached in substep S3.1, to your final set of recommendations that will appear in Act substep A1.1, the next step in the Problem-Solving Method. Anyone reading these two conclusions would expect to see the following action-oriented recommendation in Act phase substep A1.1: *Enter into a joint venture with MedSpine.*

Just like making judgments, drawing conclusions is difficult because it requires higher order thinking skills of synthesis and integration of information. You have engaged in a long process of problem study, and now must converge on a set of conclusions that distill all of your work into a set of statements that set the stage for your recommended course of action in the Act phase of the Problem-Solving Method.

STEPS TO SYNTHESIZE JUDGMENTS INTO A SET OF CONCLUSIONS

- Step 1: Review your judgments for each alternative in your problem area decision criteria table, and also work backward from those judgments and review the findings that led to those conclusions. Verify that the logic flow from your findings to your judgments is clear and convincing.
- Step 2: Review your judgments for each alternative solution and synthesize them into conclusions.
- Step 3: Review your conclusions for each alternative to see if any conclusion should be written about the alternatives relative to each other.

TIPS TO SYNTHESIZE JUDGMENTS INTO A SET OF CONCLUSIONS

■ Take the time to review and reflect on all of your work, using the working papers of tools you have created, including the stakeholder analysis table and the problem area summary table from the Define phase, through to your numbered list of findings and judgments, and your problem area decision criteria table. Does the logic flow across the steps? Are your conclusions well-supported?

■ Focus on making your conclusions as complete, yet concise, as possible. Conclusions must be understandable to anyone who reads them or hears them.

CONCLUSIONS TOOL

Review all of the tools you have completed through applying the steps of the Problem-Solving Method. Then, review your numbered lists of findings and judgments as you review your completed problem area decision criteria table. Based on the table, write a set of cogent, concise conclusions that summarize your judgments about the preferred alternatives.

Write out each of your conclusions, grouped by problem area.

ACTIVITIES TO SYNTHESIZE JUDGMENTS INTO A SET OF CONCLUSIONS

■ STUDY ACTIVITY 15

For each problem area, develop your conclusions about the alternatives based on your judgments of the pros and cons/strengths and weaknesses you have drawn about each alternative.

SUMMARY OF DEFINE AND STUDY PHASES

As a reminder, you have now worked through two waves of divergent/convergent thinking (Figure 11.2). The first wave was in the Define phase when you engaged in stakeholder interviews and identified difficulties to "make the problem bigger." Then you grouped the difficulties into problem areas to identify the key issues and converged on a problem statement and vision for the future.

Then in the Study phase you engaged in divergent thinking by brainstorming a range of possible root causes and potential alternative solutions for the difficulties in each of the problem areas. Through research, you converged on a set of conclusions that will now drive your recommendations.

These waves of divergent—convergent thinking have helped you avoid solving the wrong problem, and prevented you from jumping to recommendations that aren't

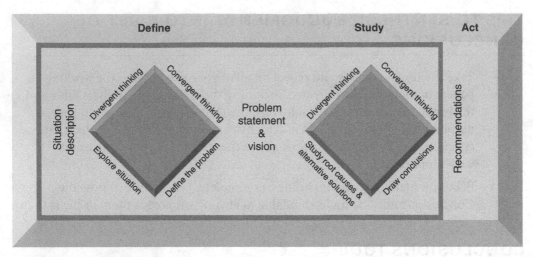

FIGURE 11.2 Two waves of divergent-convergent thinking.

addressing the true underlying root causes of the problem. You are now ready to move to the Act phase of the Problem-Solving Method. In this phase, you will state your action-oriented recommendations and focus on a communication plan to maximize the likelihood that your recommendations will be successfully implemented.

Practicing the steps of these first two phases has taken time, especially since you are writing out each step, and summarizing your logic and work in tables. As you gain experience in applying the steps, you will no longer need to write them out, and the thought process will become automatic.

REFERENCES

1. ODI. *Management techniques: force field analysis.* 2009. https://www.odi.org/publications/5218-management-techniques-force-field-analysis
2. Hammond JS, Keeney RL, Raiffa H. *Smart choices: a practical guide to making better decisions.* Boston, MA: Harvard Business Press Review; 1999.

CHAPTER 12

STUDY PHASE ACTIVITY KEY

S1.1: GENERATE POSSIBLE ROOT CAUSES (IN CHAPTER 9)

■ **STUDY ACTIVITY 1 KEY**

Generate Root Causes for the Difficulties in Each Problem Area

The Activity Key provides a brainstormed list of possible root causes for the Care Model problem area. Remember, possible root causes begin to get identified during your stakeholder analysis and other preliminary data analysis and fact finding you completed during the Define phase. You then add additional possible root causes through reading literature, talking to experts and colleagues, and brainstorming.

Care Model Difficulties

Look at the difficulties in the Care Model problem area. Then, look at those difficulties to brainstorm possible root causes. The difficulties identified in the Define Activity 14 in the Activity Key in Chapter 8 were difficulties # 5, 7, 8, 9, 10, 12, 14, and 15. They are repeated below.

5. Several stakeholders are opposed to the MedSpine joint venture solution. They believe it will hurt the hospital's volume and revenue, hurt the physical therapy department because of layoffs, and hurt the surgeons. The hospital CFO believes the service line leaders are jumping to a "terrible solution."

7. Prism Health System's costs of providing spine care are high compared to insurance industry local, regional, and national benchmarks, and are rising rapidly. The Health Plan CEO said this is making it difficult to price the Prism Health Plan's products at a competitive premium rate.

8. The Health Plan CEO said that they will be starting a Spine Center of Distinction Program, and that the Prism Health System risks not being the "right partner" for their value-based initiative that will be based on costs and outcomes of spine care.

9. The musculoskeletal service line leaders were surprised when they learned that their costs of spine care are high compared to insurance industry benchmarks.

10. The administrator reported that their internal data are incomplete, but that the service line was on track and trending upward as desired for revenue, volume, and utilization in physical therapy, musculoskeletal imaging, and surgical procedures. He did not mention cost data for the service line.

12. The newly hired spine surgeon is not convinced that the MedSpine care model is good for patients.

14. The physical therapist is opposed to bringing outsiders in to provide care, especially since she reports that Prism Health System doesn't have any protocols in place to manage patients with chronic neck and back pain.

15. The Hospital CFO says that they should be deciding the clinical care model, not the health plan.

Possible Root Causes

Here is a list of possible root causes for the difficulties listed. Remember that at this point you don't know if these are the actual root causes. You won't uncover that until you get to Study substep 2.3 as you develop findings through your research. Brainstorm as many possible root causes as you can.

1. The surgeon is providing care that is too aggressive given the patient's condition (e.g., conducting too many scans and doing surgery when it is inappropriate).

2. The spine patients seen at Prism are higher complexity, so they generate costs that are higher compared to insurance industry benchmarks because they need surgery. ("My patients are sicker.")

3. The health plan is not sharing their cost data with the health system in a structured or timely manner.

4. The hospital does not track and report cost and outcome data for treating patients with chronic neck and back pain.

5. The hospital tracks cost and outcome data, but it is not being used by the dyad leadership team.

6. Prism's compensation for surgeons and managers rewards revenue and volume production, not costs and patient outcomes.

7. Hospital personnel fear they will lose their jobs or have to lay off staff, or make changes that they believe will financially harm the hospital.

8. Prism does not have care protocols in place for treating patients with chronic neck and back pain.

9. Prism has care protocols for patients with chronic neck and back pain, but they are not being followed.

10. Prism's clinicians believe they are providing best practice care in treating patients with chronic neck and back problems.

11. Prism clinicians do not believe that non-surgical treatment for patients with chronic neck and back problems is good patient care.

12. Prism's clinicians are unaware of current best practices in treating patients with chronic neck and back problems.

13. Prism clinicians lack the expertise to provide non-surgical treatment to patients with chronic neck and back pain.

If you are the service line leaders who are using the Problem-Solving Method, as part of the "never assume" mindset, you would also want to consider the following as possible root causes:

14. As dyad leaders, we do not know how to make strategic decisions.

15. As dyad leaders, we need to improve our ability to lead the musculoskeletal service line.

■ STUDY ACTIVITY 2 KEY

As shown in Figure 12.1, the cause-effect diagram provides a way to visualize the list of possible root causes for the Care Model problem area. Note that the "Service Line Leadership" box has a grey background because as a student consulting team, this would probably be an area that you would *not* include unless you had been specifically asked by your preceptors, who are the service line leadership team.

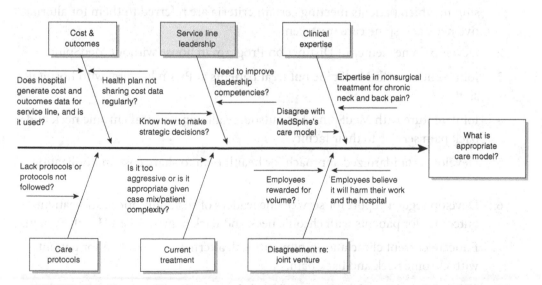

FIGURE 12.1 Cause-effect diagram of possible root causes for care model problem area.

But, if you are the service line leadership team using the Problem-Solving Method, then as part of the "never assume" mindset, this is a possible root cause that you should be considering.

S1.2: GENERATE POTENTIAL ALTERNATIVE SOLUTIONS (IN CHAPTER 9)

■ STUDY ACTIVITY 3 KEY

Solutions Preferred By Stakeholders

The following potential alternative solutions relevant for the Care Model problem area were mentioned by one or more stakeholders:

1. Do nothing – keep the status quo.
2. Develop best practice treatment protocols for managing patients with chronic neck and back pain.
3. Joint venture with MedSpine – treat patients with MedSpine staff at hospital.

■ STUDY ACTIVITY 4 KEY

Following are eight additional alternatives that provide examples of potential alternative solutions that would address the possible root causes. As you conduct your research in Study substep S2.3, you may learn about additional alternatives from the experts you interview. If so, you should come back to this step and add them to your list.

1. Do not develop a joint venture with MedSpine, but develop a referral partnership in which patients meeting certain criteria are referred to them for alternative neck and spine care treatment.
2. Develop Spine Center of Distinction Program in house without MedSpine.
3. Joint venture with MedSpine but treat patients at Prism hospital with hospital staff.
4. Joint venture with MedSpine, but outsource all non-surgical chronic neck and back pain service to their facility.
5. Develop a standardized approach for health plan to share cost and utilization data with the musculoskeletal service line.
6. Develop regular report for service line leaders of cost, utilization, and patient outcomes for patients with chronic neck and back pain at Prism Health System.
7. Educate current clinicians on non-surgical, alternative treatment for patients with chronic neck and back pain.
8. Hire new clinicians whose expertise is in non-surgical, alternative treatment for patients with chronic neck and back pain.

■ STUDY ACTIVITY 5 KEY

You may be thinking that by this step, the problem area summary table is too big to manage on a sheet of paper. Focus on using the table as an organizing tool to summarize your work, rather than something that you are trying to squeeze into one regular size sheet of paper with every single word on it.

Think of the table as an organizing structure for your work. For example, the layout works well when you are working with a team in a conference room with a large whiteboard.

Again, the point is to get into the habit of organizing and summarizing your work to support your thought process.

S2.1: DEVELOP DECISION CRITERIA (IN CHAPTER 10)

■ STUDY ACTIVITY 6 KEY

Keep in mind that Prism Health System is pursuing the Triple Aim as a strategic imperative. Thus, the decision criteria should address the criteria of the Triple Aim, in addition to other relevant decision criteria. Possible decision criteria for the Care Model problem area, and the criteria measures, might include the following:

1. Improve outcomes for patients with musculoskeletal issues—pain interfering with activities of daily living decrease by x%.
2. Patient satisfaction—increase in satisfaction scores by x% for patients with musculoskeletal issues.
3. Clinician acceptance—key stakeholders are satisfied by the alternative.
4. Total cost of care for musculoskeletal services—reduce cost to x percentile of insurance industry benchmarks.
5. Health system financial performance—x% increase in operating margin.
6. Time frame required for implementation—can it be completed in x months?
7. Training/other development costs—$.

■ STUDY ACTIVITY 7 KEY

Problem Area Decision Criteria Table

You should create one problem area decision criteria table per problem area. Thus, you would have four decision criteria tables: Care Model, Payer Relations, Goal Misalignment, and Decision-Making Model. The first row of each table should list the alternative solutions you have identified. The header of each column should list the decision criteria, as shown in Table 10.1. All other cells of the table should be blank for now.

S2.2: DETERMINE INFORMATION NEEDED (IN CHAPTER 10)

■ STUDY ACTIVITY 8 KEY

Information Needed

Based on your decision criteria for the Care Model problem area, information needed could include the questions that follow. You can see that some of the questions are seeking to uncover root causes, some are helping you better understand the current situation, and others are gathering data to judge the alternatives against the criteria.

1. What is the current community market need for musculoskeletal services for chronic neck and back pain? Volumes, percent market share that is Prism's, unmet community need, models of care provided by competitors in the marketplace?

2. If Prism entered into a joint venture with MedSpine, what are the projections for the impact on an increase in volume? In revenue generated?

3. What are the pros and cons of entering into a joint venture with MedSpine versus Prism developing and offering nontraditional care on its own? How about for the different ways of staffing the joint venture—using MedSpine's clinicians versus Prism's?

4. How are changes in reimbursement methods or models for patients with chronic neck and back pain affecting hospital revenues now and in the future? What are the coming changes, and how much could they adversely affect Prism financially if the status quo is maintained? If alternative care is provided instead of our current model of care?

5. What is Prism Health Plan's time frame for starting a Spine Center of Distinction Program? What are the parameters they will use for choosing a care delivery partner? Will we be able to fulfill those parameters in that time frame if we enter into a joint venture with MedSpine versus if we don't enter into a joint venture?

6. What are the best ways to reward clinicians and managers when reimbursement no longer pays based on volume and utilization, but value?

7. What are MedSpine's outcomes of care, and how do those outcomes compare to Prism's?

8. What are MedSpine's patient satisfaction scores, and how do they compare to Prism's?

9. What are MedSpine's costs of care, and how do they compare to Prism? Are the patients treated at MedSpine comparable in case mix/severity to Prism's?

10. Do Prism musculoskeletal service line leaders have readily available and regular access to cost and outcome data on the patients they treat? If yes, how is it made available and is it being used? If not, why not, and what would it take to provide the cost and outcome data? If Prism Health Plan has the data, what data do they have, and how might it best be shared with the Prism health system?

11. Do Prism's clinicians have the requisite knowledge to offer nontraditional care if the joint venture is not pursued? If not, how is this expertise developed and how long does that take?

12. What are Spine Center of Excellence best practices? How do Prism's and MedSpine's current treatment patterns stack up against best practices? Are Prism's clinicians aware of the best practices, and do they agree that they are best practices?

13. Does Prism currently have any protocols of best practices for treating patients with chronic neck and back pain? If not, why not? If yes, how were they developed and how are they being used?

14. What are Prism's current costs of spine care, including cost per case by diagnostic related group or outpatient code? What are the insurance industry's cost benchmarks, and at what percentile are Prism's costs?

15. Are the case mix/patient complexity of Prism's patients with musculoskeletal care needs higher than the benchmarks ("patients are sicker")? Are all comers for spine care treated at Prism, or are less severe patients deemed to not need surgery referred elsewhere?

If you are working on a real-world project, each of these questions is able to be answered through research. However, if you are working on a fictional written case, then some of these questions cannot be answered because you don't have real data. In those situations, you should talk with your mentor or an expert you are interviewing about what might be reasonable assumptions to make as answers to them.

■ STUDY ACTIVITY 9 KEY

Research Plan

The research plan should be similar to Table 10.2. For each question you identified in Activity 8, you should translate that into the information you need, where you will get it, and track progress on obtaining it.

For example, question 13 in the preceding would be summarized like the first entry in Table 10.2. You need specific cost information as summarized in the data request column, and the source is from the finance department. To expedite your request, your preceptor told you that you should submit your request through the Chief Financial Officer so that it can be moved to the front of the queue. Otherwise you may not get the information in the time frame needed to complete your project.

S2.3: DEVELOP FINDINGS THROUGH RESEARCH (IN CHAPTER 10)

■ STUDY ACTIVITY 10 KEY

Study activity 10 has no activity key associated with it, as it is instructing you to conduct an interview or read a journal article to develop findings.

■ STUDY ACTIVITY 11 KEY

Example Findings

An example of several findings for the Care Model problem area that would be summarized on your master list of findings might be similar to the ones listed in the following:

1. Prism currently has 20% of the market share for patients needing musculo-skeletal care. There are two other competitors that offer this care, and both of their websites tout their focus on non-surgical treatment for neck and back problems.

2. Based on interviews with several stakeholders, Prism has no care protocols in place for patients with chronic neck and back pain. The primary treatment mode focuses on surgery after a waiting period to see if symptoms improve. There is a lack of general awareness among clinicians of what best practices are for spine care using non-surgical methods, and Prism clinicians report that they are not trained or knowledgeable in non-surgical treatment options and approaches. According to George Stewart, head of orthopedics at HealthStar, it would take about a year for clinicians to develop their expertise in offering the non-surgical treatment approaches.

3. Interviewees' pros and cons of a joint venture versus developing our own treatment protocols and approach for nontraditional care:

   Pros of a joint venture:

   a. According to the Prism Health Plan CEO, MedSpine has extensive clinical expertise in the non-traditional clinical care process, as well as demonstrated cost and outcomes data. The peer-reviewed journal articles published by MedSpine document with well-designed clinical trials that their approach results in better patient outcomes at lower treatment cost. Interviews with the National Spine Organization's chief medical officer confirmed that MedSpine is known nationally for its cost-effective care model.

   b. The CEO of MedSpine said that because MedSpine specializes in non-surgical treatment, their care protocols are state of the art, best practice, efficient, and cost-effective. He provided results from their patient satisfaction scores that show their scores are in the top 10% over the past 3 years.

c. According to the Prism Health System COO, it would not make financial sense to engage in a partnership with MedSpine that is not a joint venture. This is because without some type of financial arrangement with them, Prism would be referring away potential patients, resulting in decreased revenue for Prism Health System. He believes it is better to enter into a formal arrangement of a joint venture with shared financial risk and reward. He said this option gets Prism Health System the clinical expertise it needs to offer best practice non-surgical care for neck and back pain with a national company that is well known and respected in the marketplace. It helps "brand" Prism Health System's musculoskeletal care to have its name associated with MedSpine.

d. (Additional findings of the pros of joint ventures would continue here.)

Cons of a joint venture:

e. The hospital staff are expressing fear of change and displacement by outsourcing. The Spine Surgeon has stated that he is not convinced that MedSpine's non-surgical approach to care is good for patients.

f. According to Laura Latter, a national joint venture expert, fear by clinicians and other staff can damage morale and harm the reputation of the hospital. She said that clinicians do not like being told what to do, especially if it is an outside organization that is coming in. She said this might be especially true if MedSpine has very specific treatment protocols that must be followed.

g. She also said that cost savings promised by joint venture outsourcing contracts are sometimes never realized. She believes that in this situation, however, it is likely that the rate of conducting surgery as a treatment option is what is driving the high costs of care. She said this is because operating room time is expensive, with high fixed costs. Thus, any treatment that drives high volume of surgery will be more expensive than non-surgical approaches. She said surgery also means longer recovery times for patients, which can limit their ability to return to work.

h. (Additional findings about cons of the joint venture would continue here.)

4. According to Prism Health System's COO and Prism Health Plan's CEO, the reimbursement model is moving from fee-for-service to a bundled payment. Under this model, health systems can share in the savings that accrue from providing cost-effective care. They said that unless Prism Health System can reduce its cost of treatment for patients with musculoskeletal issues, it will lose market share because it cannot remain cost competitive. But they said it's not just "about the money." Reimbursement changes are also paying for outcomes. It is a "value" equation.

5. According to the Prism Health Plan CEO, it is targeting a time frame of 18 to 24 months to start its Spine Center of Distinction program. It would like Prism Health System to be its clinical partner in this initiative, but the Health System will need to demonstrate its ability to provide more cost-effective care that is in line with more conservative treatment approaches that do not rely so heavily on surgery.

6. (Your list of findings summarized from your research of the remaining research questions would continue here.)

Once you have summarized your findings into a numbered list, you should populate the cells of your Problem Area Decision Table. An example completed for the decision criteria of the Care Model problem area for the two alternatives of Do Nothing and Joint Venture is shown in Table 12.1.

Remember that the purpose of creating the problem area decision table is to put your findings into a format that helps you make judgments and draw conclusions about what you have learned through your research in the Study step S3. If you are working on a student team consulting project, it is helpful to use a white board to complete this substep to facilitate discussion about the findings and how to organize them in the table.

S2.4: REVIEW, REFLECT AND REVISE APPROACH (IN CHAPTER 10)

■ STUDY ACTIVITY 12 KEY

All of the tables you have generated so far in your work are very detailed. This is too much detail to share with your preceptors. You need to refresh their memory of the problem areas and the issue and problem statements, and summarize your research conducted and findings in a way that is easily digestible for the preceptors to review and absorb during your meeting with them. Summarize your work in a few pages at most that you will share with them at the meeting.

Be prepared to discuss what you think the findings mean. That is, jumping ahead to your judgments and conclusions, Study step S3, what are the findings telling you about the pros and cons, and strengths and weaknesses of the alternatives? Which look like they are rising to the top? Is your logic sound? Do they think there are holes in your work that need further research?

Discuss with them the implications for the various stakeholders. For example, if the joint venture looks to be the best course of action, what advice do your organizational preceptors have to address the potential disagreement.

■ STUDY ACTIVITY 13 KEY

Think about what your overall goals are for the meeting with your preceptors. You want to ensure that they are supportive of work you have completed to date and what some of your preliminary thoughts are regarding your conclusions and recommendations. In

TABLE 12.1 Example Problem Area Decision Criteria Table*

CARE MODEL	PATIENT OUTCOMES	PATIENT SATISFACTION	CLINICIAN ACCEPTANCE	TOTAL COST OF CARE	HEALTH SYSTEM OPERATING MARGIN	TIME FRAME TO IMPLEMENT	COST TO IMPLEMENT
Criteria Measure	↑ by x%	↑ by x%	↑ by x%	↓ by x%	↑ by x%	< x months	< $ cost
Do Nothing-Status Quo				#1,4			
Joint Venture	#2, 3a, 3b	#3a,b	#3d, 3e	#3f, 3g	#1, 3f, 3g, 4		
Alternative Solution 3...							

*The numbers in the cells correspond to the numbered findings in the example answers in the Study Activity 11 Key provide earlier.

addition, you want to have them identify any areas where they think more research is warranted.

Remember, you do not want your organizational preceptors to be surprised by any of your work. This status meeting helps ensure that they are fully informed and in agreement with your work to date.

S3.1: COLLATE, ANALYZE, AND JUDGE THE ALTERNATIVE SOLUTIONS (IN CHAPTER 11)

■ STUDY ACTIVITY 14 KEY

Based on the example findings about the MedSpine joint venture option in the preceding Study Activity 11 Key, the following are example judgments based on those findings.

Pros/Strengths of MedSpine Joint Venture (JV) Alternative: The MedSpine JV:

1. Positions Prism Health System for the changing value-based reimbursement models; for example, bundled payments.

2. Facilitates the Health System's ability to be an attractive partner for the Prism Health Plan's Spine Center of Distinction program.

3. Enables Prism Health System to bring in the clinical expertise needed to offer non-surgical treatment protocols with published accounts of superior outcomes and high patient satisfaction for those with chronic neck and back problems.

4. Supports Prism Health System's ability to offer non-surgical treatment protocols more quickly than if it were to develop the capability in house by training their own clinicians.

Cons/Weaknesses of MedSpine Joint Venture (JV) Alternative:

5. The MedSpine JV is feared and opposed by many clinicians and some managers in the hospital, and might harm the hospital's reputation if this opposition is made public.

6. The spine surgeon does not believe the MedSpine care model is helpful for his patients, and as a key stakeholder, could greatly hinder the hospital's ability to implement and sustain the care model.

7. Because the hospital currently has no treatment protocols for treating patients with chronic neck and back pain, its culture may not support protocol-based treatment models. Yet, success with the joint venture will require adherence to treatment protocols. Clinicians may feel that this stifles their autonomy.

Based on your numbered list, the row that lists the joint venture as the alternative solution would list the following in its "Your Judgment" column: Pros: # 1 to 4; Cons: # 5 to 7.

S3.2: SYNTHESIZE JUDGMENTS INTO A SET OF CONCLUSIONS

■ STUDY ACTIVITY 15 KEY

An example conclusion that could be drawn from the findings and judgments provided earlier about the joint venture option is:

> *The MedSpine joint venture option is well aligned with the changing reimbursement models that drive value over volume, and Prism Health System's commitment to the cost, quality, and access goals of the Triple Aim. MedSpine's published clinical trials have documented cost-effective care with superior patient outcomes and high patient satisfaction with their non-surgical approaches to treating chronic neck and back pain.*

In your research, you likely reviewed the cost data to determine the financial impact the joint venture would have on the hospital financially. You would need to provide a conclusion about what the financial impact might be short-term and long-term, and why the joint venture option is still a preferable option.

You can't just sugarcoat the joint venture option conclusions; you also have to document logic of what the downsides of the joint venture are, but why it still remains a preferred alternative.

Finally, if there are others who completed the activities in these chapters, compare your conclusions to theirs. What are the strengths of the different conclusions? How might some of them be reworded to make them stronger, more concise, and more convincing?

You now have worked through all of the steps in the Define and Study phases, and are ready to move on to practice the Act phase of the Problem-Solving Method in Part IV of the text.

PART IV

DEFINE

D1. Situation & Scope	D2. Stakeholders, Difficulties, & Problem Areas	D3. Issue Statements & Problem Statement
D1.1 Describe the *situation* D1.2 Scope the work	D2.1 Begin stakeholder analysis D2.2 Identify *difficulties* D2.3 Group difficulties into *problem areas*	D3.1 Create *issue statement* for each problem area D3.2 Create overall *problem statement* and vision for future

STUDY

S1. Root Causes & Alternative Solutions	S2. Decision Criteria, Research, & Findings	S3. Conclusions
S1.1 Generate possible root causes S1.2 Generate potential alternative solutions	S2.1 Develop decision criteria S2.2 Determine additional information needed S2.3 Develop *findings* through research S2.4 Review, reflect, and revise approach	S3.1 Collate, analyze, and judge the alternative solutions S3.2 Synthesize judgments into a set of *conclusions*

ACT

A1. Recommendations & Milestones	A2. Communication Strategy & Consensus Building	A3. Implementation & Monitoring
A1.1 Create integrated set of *recommendations* A1.2 Develop key implementation milestones	A2.1 Revisit stakeholder analysis A2.2 Create communication plan A2.3 Implement communication plan and validate approval/consensus of recommendations	A3.1 Develop detailed implementation plan A3.2 Monitor results against key performance indicators

PRACTICE THE ACT PHASE

OVERVIEW OF PART IV

Part IV of the text provides the "how-to" practice chapters for the Act phase to help you learn each of the steps in this phase. There is one practice chapter per step (Chapters 13, 14, and 15), followed by the answer key for the practice activities in each of the of Study phase chapters (Chapter 16). All of your work in the Act phase builds on your work in the Define and Study phases, so Chapters 5 through 11 must be completed before you progress to Chapters 13 through 15.

The structure of each practice chapter is as follows:

- A brief overview of the step and its substeps
- The "how-to" of completing each substep
- Key steps to complete each substep
- Tips for completing each substep successfully
- Tools that support writing up your work in each substep
- Activities for you to practice each substep

As you work your way through the "how-to" practice chapters, it will be very helpful for you to go back to Chapter 2 to read its corresponding detailed information regarding the "what" description for each Act phase substep.

Many of the activities use The Spinal Frontier case in Chapter 1 for you to practice the Problem-Solving Method. The Activity Key chapter provides answers or suggested responses based on The Spinal Frontier case.

As you complete each chapter, you will complete a written product for each of the substeps in it. Thus, practice chapters should be completed in order, because the work you complete in each practice chapter is used in the next one. Writing out your work is important for internalizing the Problem Solving Method. As you gain experience in using the Method, you will rarely write out the step; they will instead be a part of your logical thought process.

Leave yourself time for uninterrupted attention to work through each chapter. The activities will require your thoughtful application.

CHAPTER 13

PRACTICE ACT STEP A1: RECOMMENDATIONS AND MILESTONES

OVERVIEW OF ACT PHASE

Based on the work you completed in the Define and Study phases, you are now ready to begin practicing the Act phase. Part IV of the text covers the Act phase, shown in Figure 13.1. It is comprised of three steps, each of which has two or more substeps:

A1: Recommendations and Milestones (Chapter 13)

A2: Communication Strategy and Consensus Building (Chapter 14)

A3: Implementation and Monitoring (Chapter 15)

It is in the Act phase that your conclusions for each problem area get integrated into one holistic set of recommendations for the problem. You then identify the major steps that would be required to implement your recommendations so that the stakeholders who will be consenting to or approving your recommendation have an idea of the resources required by your recommendations.

You next focus on your communication strategy, paying particular attention to your presentation to the key stakeholders who will be voting on or consenting to your recommendations. Once approved, you need to develop a detailed implementation plan with a set of key performance indicators that will be used to monitor results.

The structure of the Act phase practice chapters is identical to that of the Define and Study phases. Each substep begins with a brief overview and a "how-to" description section, followed by the steps, tips, tools and activities. As you work through these "how-to" practice chapters, remember to refer back to Chapter 2 for the in-depth "what" description of each step and substep.

Chapter 16 contains the Activity Key example answers for the activities found in the three practice chapters for the Act phase.

When you have completed the Act phase, you will have developed a set of action-oriented recommendations and strategically communicated them to key stakeholders and decision makers for approval or consensus. The recommendations will have a set of key implementation milestones as well as a detailed implementation plan.

Act

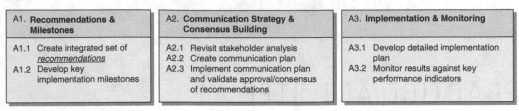

FIGURE 13.1 Act phase of the Problem-Solving Method.

ACT STEP A1: RECOMMENDATIONS AND MILESTONES

As shown in Figure 13.2, there are two substeps in the recommendations and milestone step in the Act phase of the Problem-Solving Method: A1.1, Create integrated set of recommendations; and A1.2, Develop key implementation milestones.

PRACTICE A1.1: CREATE INTEGRATED SET OF RECOMMENDATIONS

*Recommendations are an integrated set of **action-oriented** solutions that answer the questions posed in the issue statements and problem statements while simultaneously heading the organization toward its vision for the future.*

HOW TO CREATE AN INTEGRATED SET OF RECOMMENDATIONS

Action-oriented recommendations are the final set of preferred alternative solutions based on your conclusions across *all* of the problem areas. Begin each recommendation with an action verb. List your primary recommendations first. If the situation calls for both short-term and long-term recommendations, the sequence and timing of the recommendations should be clear. Recommendations should be stated succinctly, and it should be clear what action is being requested. They should be consistent across each other, and as an integrated set, resolve the root causes of the difficulties, closing the gap between "what is" and "what ought to be" to solve the problem as defined.

ACT

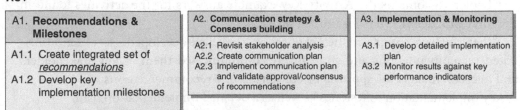

FIGURE 13.2 Act step A1: Recommendations and milestones.

KEY STEPS TO CREATE AN INTEGRATED SET OF RECOMMENDATIONS

Step 1: Review the problem area decision criteria table and collate the alternative solutions that were judged to be acceptable.

Step 2: For each alternative solution accepted across all problem areas, develop an action-oriented recommendation.

Step 3: Synthesize the recommendations into a set that lays out a high-level plan of action for the organization.

Step 4: Organize the set of recommendations from the most impactful and cascade the other recommendations to support the efforts of the most important recommendations.

TIPS TO CREATE AN INTEGRATED SET OF RECOMMENDATIONS

- The actions stated in the recommendations should be at a high level. If they contain detail of when, where, and who, they are becoming too detailed. This level of detail should be included only in the milestones or implementation plan.

- If there are issues in the problem that must be resolved immediately, be sure that your recommendations for those issues can be implemented immediately. Students and early careerists often underestimate the time it takes to implement change. When in doubt, talk with mentors and industry contacts about reasonable time frames for how long it might take to get your recommendations implemented.

- Your set of recommendations should be listed logically, either from short-term to long-term, or most important to least important. Avoid simply providing a list of recommendations in random order.

A few recommendations are listed in the following in Act Activity 1. You will notice they are listed randomly. A set of recommendations should look different than the list that follows. They should cascade by categories such as order of implementation, by importance, by stakeholder, and so on. Additionally, the recommendation statements should be listed one recommendation at a time. Comingling two ideas becomes confusing for the audience and will be difficult once you move to the presentation strategy step.

RECOMMENDATIONS TOOL

As you develop your recommendations, you should have in front of you your numbered lists of findings and judgments, and your problem area decision criteria table. Once you have written your recommendations, you should go back to the problem area summary table to review your problem statement and vision for the future. Then look at the set of recommendations you have created to ensure they are answering the questions posed in the problem statement, and that if successfully implemented, will help the organization move toward its vision for the future.

ACTIVITIES TO CREATE AN INTEGRATED SET OF RECOMMENDATIONS

■ ACT ACTIVITY 1

Review the set of recommendations that follow for The Spinal Frontier case. Decide on a category that will effectively help explain the recommendations in an integrated set. Arrange the recommendations by this category. Add any additional recommendations that are missing from your analysis and arrange these in the category. As a reminder, categories to consider are by timeline (e.g., short-term vs. long-term), importance, stakeholder, or other categories you can determine that make sense.

1. Prism Health should proceed with the joint venture to establish a MedSpine program at Westport Hospital

2. The steering group should have authority and should include directors from Neurosurgery, Orthopedics, Sports Medicine, Physical Therapy, and Occupational Therapy.

3. Prism Health should approach Prism Health Plan and create a Spine Center of Excellence Program.

4. The structure and role of the Prism Musculoskeletal Clinical Service Line (PMCSL) needs to be re-defined.

5. In the existing world of value-based care, PMCSL should have clear clinical protocols in place to screen and treat patients with spine issues.

■ ACT ACTIVITY 2

Think ahead to the presentation strategy step. What visuals or frameworks come to mind when looking at the recommendations as a whole? Review diagrammer.com or PowerPoint SmartArt to see if any frameworks come to mind.

PRACTICE A1.2: DEVELOP KEY IMPLEMENTATION MILESTONES

Key implementation milestones articulate at a high level the overall timelines and accountability of your recommendations.

HOW TO DEVELOP KEY IMPLEMENTATION MILESTONES

Decision makers who approve your recommendations must understand the financial and resource obligations that implementation will place on the organization. Those who will be involved in implementing the solution must fully understand their role and the major steps they must take to fulfill their obligations. This step does not require a detailed project implementation work plan, but rather the key implementation milestones with enough information for stakeholders to understand the commitment that is being made by them and the organization if the recommendations are to be implemented.

KEY STEPS TO DEVELOP KEY IMPLEMENTATION MILESTONES

Step 1: Review your recommendations to determine the order needed to implement them, and their overall timing for execution.

Step 2: Create a Gantt chart that shows the key milestones of the recommendations.

Step 3: Establish overall accountability for the major steps through identifying specific leaders or teams that will be accountable and responsible to move the specific recommendation forward.

TIPS TO DEVELOP KEY IMPLEMENTATION MILESTONES

- A Gantt chart is a bar chart used in project management. It shows the key milestones that need to be completed on the left-hand side of the chart, with a timeline along the top. The bar length for each task shows the start and end dates of the task, and the length of the bar indicates how long each task takes to complete. See www.gantt.com/ for an example.

TOOL TO DEVELOP KEY IMPLEMENTATION MILESTONES

Figure 13.3 shows an example Gantt chart that would be used to create a summary of the key milestones for implementing your recommendations.

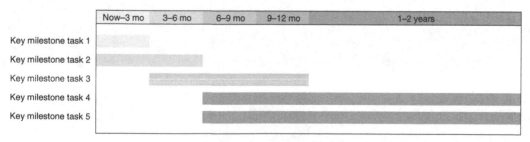

FIGURE 13.3 Example Gantt chart of key milestones.

ACTIVITIES TO DEVELOP KEY IMPLEMENTATION MILESTONES

■ ACT ACTIVITY 3

Create a Gantt chart of the key milestones for your recommendations for The Spinal Frontier case. Remember to focus on the major milestones and not on implementation detail.

CHAPTER 14

PRACTICE ACT STEP A2: COMMUNICATION STRATEGY AND CONSENSUS BUILDING

ACT STEP A2: COMMUNICATION STRATEGY AND CONSENSUS BUILDING

As shown in Figure 14.1, there are three substeps in the Communication Strategy and Consensus Building step in the Act phase of the Problem-Solving Method: A2.1, Revisit stakeholder analysis; A2.2, Create communication plan; and A2.3, Implement communication plan and validate approval/consensus of recommendations.

Remember to go back to Chapter 2 to read the "what" of Step A2 before starting the practice of the "how" in this chapter.

One of the most important aspects of Act step A2 is the presentation strategy in substep A2.3. Thus, a majority of the content in this chapter is devoted to the presentation.

PRACTICE A2.1: REVISIT STAKEHOLDER ANALYSIS

Revisit the stakeholder analysis to ensure you have a clear understanding of the various stakeholders' points of view of your recommendations, both positive and negative, so that you can develop a communications plan that builds consensus for and mitigates any resistance to the recommendations.

HOW TO REVISIT THE STAKEHOLDER ANALYSIS

At this step, circle back and revisit your stakeholder analysis to ensure you have a clear understanding of the various points of view about your recommendations and the champions and detractors of your efforts. This enables you to anticipate possible scenarios of how certain individuals or groups may respond to the recommendations. Revisiting the stakeholder analysis informs the communications plan you will develop in the next step.

Act

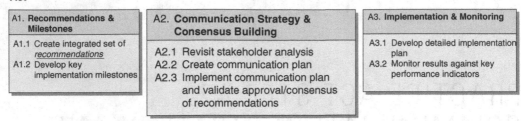

FIGURE 14.1 Act step A2: Communication strategy and consensus building.

KEY STEPS TO REVISIT THE STAKEHOLDER ANALYSIS

Step 1: From the stakeholder analysis, identify those individuals and groups that will likely be supportive of the recommendations versus those that may be hesitant and/or opposed.

Step 2: Anticipate scenarios and create contingencies where there is a possibility that the current recommendations are still not acceptable to certain stakeholders.

TIPS TO REVISIT STAKEHOLDER ANALYSIS

1. Meet with those that support the plan and confirm their support before any meetings that include a proposal presentation and/or vote. Ask these supporters to voice their endorsement during the meeting.

2. Determine if meeting directly with stakeholders still opposing the proposal would be helpful. Many times it is another supporter that may help mitigate opposition. For instance, if there is a surgeon opposed to the proposal and there is a different surgeon in agreement, perhaps the best way to gain support is for the supportive surgeon to be in the meeting with the surgeon that is opposing.

TOOL TO REVISIT STAKEHOLDER ANALYSIS

You will refer back to the stakeholder analysis table that you started in substep D2.1 of the Define phase, and updated as you worked through the Define and Study phases.

ACTIVITIES TO REVISIT THE STAKEHOLDER ANALYSIS

■ ACT ACTIVITY 4

Suppose one of your recommendations is to move forward with the MedSpine joint venture.

Which stakeholders might be opposed to that recommendation?

What scenario or contingency might you put in place, and to what end?

PRACTICE A2.2: CREATE A COMMUNICATION PLAN

A communication plan identifies the key stakeholder groups with whom you need to communicate, and the overall objective, message, format, and time frame for communicating with them, all of which may vary by stakeholder.

HOW TO CREATE THE COMMUNICATION PLAN

The communication plan lays out the considerations and steps that will be needed to gain approval or consensus of the recommendations. This step focuses on the goals of communicating with the various stakeholders, along with the who, what, when, where, and how that is needed to move the recommendations forward. The communications plan does *not* focus on the detail of the implementation steps once the recommendations are approved. In other words, the focus is on achieving consensus before the implementation begins. The communication plan should be considered well before actually presenting the information.

As you progress into future projects and your career, you will likely start your communication plan at the beginning of the project, identifying the who, what, when, and where of your communication plan and what needs to occur throughout the project. For instance, you may have a communication point, or meeting, with key stakeholders to review the major difficulties and agree on your problem areas.

Another typical point to communicate is around the alternative solution selection and, finally, any major presentation development. For most projects, your communication plan will start early in the problem-solving process and run throughout the project. In your scope of work with the project or client, you will determine up-front the key communication points needed throughout the project. It will become clearer throughout the project as to where there will be resistance and where there will be support. As these develop, conversations and meetings should be occurring to ensure that the final presentation or step will result in the plan's approval.

KEY STEPS TO CREATE THE COMMUNICATION PLAN

Step 1: List the goals of the communication plan. Identify the stakeholder groups from whom you and your team need the approval of your recommendations—such as the Board of Directors, Capital or Finance Committees, City Council, County Commissions to go through Business Planning Processes, approval of your executive team, director, manager, and so forth. Identify what level of approval is needed by which stakeholders to move the recommendations forward; for example, a formal vote versus consensus only versus information only.

Step 2: For each stakeholder group, determine the message that needs to be communicated and what format will be most effective to communicate it. Examples include a formal presentation, written report, email, press conference/press statement, press release, phone call, or an in-person conversation. Additionally, you will want to develop a plan for what, how, and who will communicate the message and when it will occur. If it is a meeting, you need to be clear about the participants who should be in the room.

Step 3: Review the stakeholder analysis again to determine if there are any among these groups who may not be supportive of the recommendations and if so, implications for the communication plan.

Step 4: Begin developing your communication plan materials; for example, draft Power-Point presentations, emails, and so on. Work with administrative staff or project managers to schedule meetings.

TIPS TO CREATE THE COMMUNICATION PLAN

- Consider the purpose of the meeting—what do you hope to accomplish? The opening remarks of any presentation should grab the audience's attention and also include the end goal of the meeting, whether it is consensus on an issue or a formal vote to implement the recommendations.

- Carefully plan the *strategy* of the presentation. It need not be in the same order as the written report, and in fact, it probably should not be. Think about the best way to *sell* the recommendations to the decision makers present at the gathering.

- Know the time constraints and the scope of what can be accomplished during the meeting. This may include presenting all of the issues or only the top three.

- Know the audience. Does it include the Board, the CEO, physicians, members of the community or the media, your boss? Make sure the key people who support your recommendations will be there. What information will be critical to this audience when considering the recommendations? What details are appropriate for the level of your audience? Some stakeholders may be more focused on cost-effectiveness, others on patient experience. Understand what aspects appeal to each stakeholder and plan your points accordingly.

- Understand the time frame of the problem and your recommendations. Is the problem short term or long term? Is your audience prepared to act on all of your recommendations at the meeting, or only some of them?

- Think through what questions you may get asked and by whom, and how you will answer them. Think about how to handle points of debate with respect and anticipate the different viewpoints of your audience. Answer questions objectively with regard to what's best for the organization. Do not interpret challenging questions as personal attacks on you. Be confident that you can answer the hard questions.

TOOL TO CREATE THE COMMUNICATION PLAN

Table 14.1 shows an example table to outline the communication plan. In the first column you list the stakeholders with whom you need to communicate and what their role

TABLE 14.1 Communication Plan

GOALS	DESCRIPTION AND DETAILS OF FORUM + ATTENDEES	WHAT IS THE KEY FOCUS FOR THE AUDIENCE	IN WHAT FORMAT WILL THE INFORMATION BE COMMUNICATED	WHO WILL COMMUNICATE INFORMATION	STAKEHOLDER AGREEMENT/ DISCERNMENT NOTES
Board Approval					
Executive Team Approval					
Capital Resource Planning Committee Approval					
Full-Time Equivalent Resource Team Approval					
Physician Buy-In					
RN Staff Buy-In					
Other Staff Awareness					
Community Awareness or Formal Approval (Certified Nursing Assistant, Building, etc.)					
Positive Media Coverage					
Other					

is (e.g., formal approval vs. buy-in vs. awareness). The next columns summarize the remainder of the plan—what is the forum for the communication and who will be there, what is the key message for that audience and how will it be communicated, who is the right person to do the communicating, and how might the stakeholders respond to the message.

ACTIVITIES TO CREATE THE COMMUNICATION PLAN

Continue using The Spinal Frontier case from Chapter 1 as you complete these activities.

■ ACT ACTIVITY 5

Create a communication plan for the project preceptors and for the steering committee noted in the case.

PRACTICE A2.3: IMPLEMENT THE COMMUNICATION PLAN AND VALIDATE APPROVAL/CONSENSUS OF RECOMMENDATIONS

Implement the communication plan via presentations and other methods in the plan to gain approval and consensus of the recommendations.

HOW TO IMPLEMENT THE COMMUNICATION PLAN AND VALIDATE APPROVAL/CONSENSUS OF RECOMMENDATIONS

Implementing the communication plan involves at least one or more formal presentations to various stakeholders who either need to vote on the recommendations or build consensus to move them forward. Additionally, the communication plan could include a written report that includes detailed information and analysis for organizations to refer to as they consider the proposal and move the project forward to implementation.

This step requires strong synthesis, presentation skills, writing skills, meeting management techniques, emotional intelligence to "read" your audience while you are presenting, and strong project management skills. You will use your communication plan as a guide to ensure the steps are carefully executed upon and no stakeholder viewpoint is left unaddressed.

■ CONTENT DEVELOPMENT

In general, not all of the information you have collected, analyzed, and synthesized to date will be audience-ready for consumption. There is another level of synthesis and ordering that needs to occur in order to effectively discuss and gain approval of the recommendations and to determine next steps.

Your work to date interviewing, reviewing data, and summarizing your work in tables are your "working papers." The information will be too detailed for stakeholders to consume in its entirety. The analogy is sharing a full Excel spreadsheet versus consolidating the data into consumable data visuals that tell a story for the audience. The same is true of the qualitative and quantitative data you have collected to date. A story needs to be told that has a well-developed logic trail and a document(s) for stakeholders and audiences to easily consume.

Some could argue that it is impossible to articulate the answer to "how should I present the information?" as you will need to know the audience to gauge the answer to this. However, there are various parameters that will assist in your presentation strategy that are listed in the following.

For those not familiar with the problem-solving terminology, it will be important to remove problem area terminology in your content. You will transform your "working papers" from the Define, Study, and Act phases into a convincing verbal and/or written deliverable that takes your different audiences into consideration, as you have outlined in the communication plan. For example, you likely would not call your problem areas, problem areas—instead you may end up organizing your presentation around key themes and outline your major questions for each theme, which are in problem-solving lingo, issue statements.

As you have discovered when creating your communication plan for Prism Health System, not all audiences will receive the same information. Remember, this is a persuasion presentation and the audience perspectives need to be considered. This is a critical part of the presentation strategy step and should be carefully considered in your communication plan, even as you are working on the Define and Study phases.

If a verbal presentation and a leave-behind document are included in your communication strategy, it is likely that you will think about two deliverable formats, the "deck" and the "doc." A deck is meant to serve as a 15 to 20 minute executive level summary presentation formatted in a PowerPoint. The doc is a more detailed deliverable, likely used for a pre-read or leave-behind. The doc could be a stand-alone PowerPoint, Word Document, or documents with written information with visuals, like a pamphlet or content website. Another format would be to combine the deck and doc, where you verbally present the deck and the appendix serves as the more detailed doc, to answer questions during the presentation or for pre-read, leave-behind purposes. Beyond the "deck" and the "doc," other formats that are commonly used that would highlight points in the process for some stakeholder audiences include the SBAR (see Chapter 5) and an A3 (see Chapter 3) described earlier in the text.

Of course every situation is different, and it is important to establish what is needed by the audiences in your communication plan. There may be times where no handout, visual guides, or written documents are appropriate; this needs to be gauged by situation and audience. Although, in general, if working on a student consulting project or a complex problem with multiple stakeholders, it is likely that both a "deck" and a "doc" will serve the communication strategy well.

As you develop your content in various formats, it can be very effective to review the material through the lens of Aristotle's Rhetorical Triangle: Logos, Ethos, and Pathos.[1] This means that you persuade through logic, author credibility, and appealing to audience emotions. The rhetorical triangle can be particularly helpful as a guidepost when developing content and your presentation document and talking points to ensure that you are presenting as credible and logical and with heart.

- Logos—Is your thought process clear in your presentation? Does your logic make sense? Are your findings credible? Is the flow of the presentation clear?

- Ethos—Is your presentation style polished and professional? Is your tone, diction, and language appropriate for the audience? Do you demonstrate respect for multiple viewpoints? Are you viewed as credible and ethical by your audience?

- Pathos—Do you provide vivid examples and images that appeal to the audience's imagination and emotions? Do you appeal to the audience's values and beliefs by using stories and scenarios they can relate to?

A complementary framework to consider while organizing your information into the "deck" or "doc" is the storytelling framework that divides content into a beginning, middle, and end. Throughout the storytelling journey, you will use contrast to crystalize major points around "what is" versus "what could be," or what we call the contrast between the difficulties and the recommendations. See the tips that follow for an outline representation of what is described in the next few paragraphs.

Beginning

The goal of the beginning of a story is to set a common understanding of the current situation. As you develop a deck or give a presentation, you will cover enough to bring all to a common understanding of the situation, scope of work, problem areas, and vision for the future. You will likely cover the importance of the topic in the context of the organization and healthcare, as well as introduce your team and cover your project approach.

Middle

The middle of a story is where the exploration of challenges and difficulties occurs. In this section, your problem areas become the backbone of the presentation and the content is around the difficulties, findings, and conclusions. As you explore each problem area, or theme if you prefer to not use problem-solving lingo, you will want to explain what is and contrast this with what could be in the future. Between the current and future state imagined, you "sprinkle" your findings to persuade the audience toward change. This includes evidence, interviews, and patient stories to build your case for change.

End

The end of the story is where the "hero emerges"—the vision set forth in the beginning comes to fruition. The last part of the presentation gives a comprehensive view of the recommendations and key milestones and usually wraps up with the vision for the future and a call to action.

■ MEETING PREPARATION

After you have developed the communication plan and the various meeting materials, there are additional steps needed to prepare for the meetings. Some areas to consider are as follows.

It is important to understand the meeting attendees and audience. Know who the chairperson is and the people in the room and understand how the group behaves. For instance, is the meeting formal and does the meeting use Robert's Rules of Order? Or is the meeting more informal and the group pursues consensus for decision-making? If you can attend a meeting before the date you will be presenting, this can help you and your team understand the format of the meetings and its attendees.

After fully understanding the meeting environment and attendees, you will stage your meeting. Staging the meeting includes reserving the room for the presentation, determining the most effective arrangement for the room, developing the agenda and the materials to be distributed, arranging for the technology that will be needed and ensuring that you know how it works prior to the meeting, and ordering food. If the meeting owner is another person or team, you will still want to check on all of these items to ensure you understand the details.

If the meeting and agenda is not set already by the team to whom you are presenting, make sure to prepare an agenda. The agenda is a guide on major points to ensure you stay within the time frame allotted. This helps with your credibility and the logic of the presentation. You will need to decide or try to influence the order of your presentation on the agenda. Would it be helpful to go first, in the middle, or last on the agenda for any particular reason? How much time is allotted for you on the agenda? All of these points may help you establish if you should present an oral presentation only while seated versus a formal PowerPoint presentation, or what type of handout would be most appropriate. You will also want to know if you need to send materials ahead of time and what kind of materials. Some meetings have a pre-read packet that is separate from the meeting packet and each set of materials may have different deadlines.

Your handouts or presentation should contain the information you deem is critical to achieving your goals for the meeting. Do not overwhelm meeting attendees with volumes and volumes of handouts or slides that are not related to the logic of your presentation. If you are voting on recommendations, distribute a written copy of the recommendations for further study before conducting the vote.

Other points you want to consider concern your presence in the meeting. What is the set-up of the room? Who will be sitting where and will you sit or stand when you present? What kind of technology is available, and do you know how to use it? What is your backup plan in the event that the technology does not work as intended during your presentation?

■ MEETING MANAGEMENT AND PRESENTATION

Regardless of the presentation format, as you present your material there are some key points you will want to consider around your audience and how you present the information. You will want to catch the audience or meeting attendees' attention up front by stating the purpose of the presentation and what you will be asking for at the end of the meeting. For instance, are you proposing a vote, a decision based on consensus, or is the meeting informational only in nature. Additionally, do not assume the audience remembers the topic at hand and why it is important. Make sure to recap the situation and background. Do not skip the beginning of the story, although do not make it so long that the audience's attention and engagement wanes.

As you are drawing the audience into the situation and begin to transition to the middle of your presentation, make sure to use facts and evidence or call out when you are restating opinions of stakeholder groupings. Be objective and show that you have asked difficult questions in your quest to solve the problem.

As you begin to answer questions, you will have anticipated many based on the work you have done to date. When answering, avoid stating "that is a great question." The reason for this is because when you do not say "great question" for the next question, your statement becomes a judgment. Instead, you could state, "Thank you for your question" or "We considered that and would like to share our thoughts as follows...." When answering questions, you should also avoid saying things like "As I stated in the presentation," or "As I just said in my answer to...." These phrases make it sound as if you are criticizing the person asking the question. Regarding questions and answers, avoid becoming defensive or judging a question as a "bad question." As you discovered in your stakeholder analysis, people come from different perspectives and it is important to be professional and respectful, even if someone else asked the same questions just a moment ago or you covered the information in your presentation.

As you are seeking consensus or discussing a vote, know what is essential in your plan versus where you and your team may be able to be flexible and modify the plan. You should have thought about these contingencies prior to the meeting. For instance, can the timing of the recommendations be adjusted, or can a subset of the recommendations be implemented as a way to test the concept? Be as flexible as you can when positive suggestions are made. Additionally, be confident. Do not say, "Well, I guess that is okay." Instead find a way to state your appreciation and show confidence in how the edit to your plan brings forward a better plan and adds value.

As the meeting closes, summarize and create action. If you are in a meeting with the Board of Directors, the Board Chair should do this. If the meeting is with the Executive Team, the Chair of the meeting should summarize to create the action. You should meet with the Meeting Chair prior to the meeting to discuss this. If the Chair does not step in and summarize the actions as expected, you should be prepared to step in to provide a summary that drives consensus or a call for a vote.

■ PRESENTATION STYLE

It is important to develop your own presentation style. Speak slowly and clearly, and don't read a speech or lecture to the audience. Use humor appropriately if you can. Let the audience see that you are prepared and confident about your analysis and recommendations through your content, although also through your pacing, tone of voice, calm demeanor and "never assume" mindset. Dress appropriately for the audience, determine if and where you will be sitting or standing before the meeting, and practice, practice, practice.

Professionalism

Remember that anything written down or said can be shared with all parties not in the room. Handouts, videos, and pictures can be distributed in an instant. Be aware of this as you choose your language when presenting, writing, finalizing handouts, and answering questions. It is very important to not make your boss or others in the room look bad. Some of the difficulties and problem areas you are addressing in your presentations may be because others have not done their job well. It is not productive to call attention to this fact during the meeting. Rather, focus on how the problem can be resolved and rely on your issue statements to ask questions that drive action versus placing blame on individuals.

KEY STEPS TO IMPLEMENT THE COMMUNICATION PLAN AND VALIDATE APPROVAL/CONSENSUS OF RECOMMENDATIONS

Step 1: Review the communication plan and engage those that will assist in carrying out the plan.

Step 2: Schedule meetings and add your project topic to standing meeting agendas.

Step 3: Create and route drafts of the presentation to those assisting in the presentation as you prepare for the meeting.

Step 4: Distribute materials according to organizational norms prior to the meeting; for example, 1 week prior to the meeting.

Step 5: Review the stakeholder agreement/disagreement from the communication plan and prepare accordingly.

Step 6: Attend the meeting, present your material, and follow-up as decided upon in the meeting.

TABLE 14.2 Example Presentation or Write-up Outline

BEGINNING	MIDDLE	END

1. Brief Description of Situation and Background
2. Overall Problem Statement and Vision for the Future
	3. List of Problem Areas, Issue Statements
	4. Problem Area 1
	  a. Main Difficulties
	  b. Alternative Solutions and Conclusions
	  c. Recommendations
	5. Problem Area 2
	  a. Main Difficulties
	  b. Alternative Solutions & Conclusions
	  c. Recommendations
	6. Repeat for All Problem Areas - same structure as 4 and 5
	7. Overall Description of Major Recommendations
	8. Implementation Consideration (Time, Money, etc)
		9. Call to Action – The Ask
		10. Vision for the Future

TIPS TO IMPLEMENT THE COMMUNICATION PLAN AND VALIDATE APPROVAL/CONSENSUS OF RECOMMENDATIONS

It can be difficult as a novice to determine how to translate all of your work into a presentation or written document that demonstrates the logic of your problem-solving project without using problem-solving lingo. Table 14.2 is an outline to consider. Remember, you generally should not use The Problem-Solving Method terminology as you present your information. The outline considers the rhetorical triangle and general storytelling outline, as discussed earlier in the chapter.

"Deck" and "Doc" Design:

- Utilize the organization's presentation templates, if they have one available. If not, use the colors of the organization with a dark gray or white background.

- Design the master slides to be consistent throughout; use only a maximum of three fonts in the slide deck if you are creating a new template.

- Use photos and icons in the presentation, and limit wordy slides. Photos are usually found within the organization's marketing department. Otherwise, be careful with copyright.

- Use time saver graphics and models (see Table 14.3 for links).

- When discussing data, avoid detailed charts. Instead note the point of the data or the takeaways.

- There should be one main idea per slide—it is best not to commingle major problem areas or major recommendations.

- Consider using an outline tracker at the top or bottom of your slides to show where you are in the presentation.

TABLE 14.3 Useful Presentation Tool and Template Websites

PRESENTATION AND DESIGN TOOL	WEBSITE
Slide Design and Storytelling	Slideology https://www.duarte.com/books/slideology
Slide Design and Slide Templates	Timesaver https://www.slideshare.net/kaurapuuro/timesaver-ppt-jk
Visuals, Diagrams, and & Icons	Noun Project https://thenounproject.com Flat Icon https://www.flaticon.com Diagrammer https://diagrammer.duarte.com

TOOLS TO IMPLEMENT THE COMMUNICATION PLAN AND VALIDATE APPROVAL/CONSENSUS OF RECOMMENDATIONS

■ DESIGN TOOLS

Table 14.3 has website links that provide useful tools and templates for developing presentations.

■ PRACTICE AND EVALUATION TOOLS

Exhibit 14.1 provides a number of useful points on which to evaluate yourself or your team as you prepare for and practice your presentation. If you are preparing for a case competition presentation, the competition will usually have a similar tool that outlines the criteria on which your team will be evaluated. Review the case competition's judging criteria to use as you develop your presentation and practice it.

ACTIVITIES TO IMPLEMENT THE COMMUNICATION PLAN AND VALIDATE APPROVAL/CONSENSUS OF RECOMMENDATIONS

■ ACT ACTIVITY 6

Prepare a PowerPoint presentation for Prism Health System. Those attending will be your preceptors (the Dyad leadership team of the Musculoskeletal Clinical Service Line), the CEO and COO of Prism Health System, the CEO of the Prism Health Plan, the hospital CFO, the Spine Surgeon, the Director of Physical Therapy, and others on the Musculoskeletal Clinical Service Line advisory group.

EXHIBIT 14.1

EXAMPLE PRESENTATION CRITERIA

I. PRESENTATION CONTENT	II. PRESENTATION DELIVERY
(Check all that apply)	(Check all that apply)
• Information organized clearly • Appropriate level of detail • Presenter(s) exhibited a deep understanding of topic • Contrast in information (i.e., problem/solution, pain/gain, before/after, etc.) • Considered target audience and was culturally sensitive • Recommendations were feasible/actionable and supported by evidence • Clear call to action and/or conclusion • Presenter(s) connected to audience's ethos (used metaphors, compelling statistic, patient story, etc.)	• Good posture and body language • Gestures were natural and comfortable (free of fidgeting) • Presentation tone is pleasant to audience and words are enunciated • Appropriate word choice • Few filler words (i.e., "um," "like," "so") • Appropriate eye contact • Appropriate dress • Transitions between team members were smooth (if applicable) • Audience was drawn to speaker(s) • Appropriate energy level (manages excitability, although keeps energy up) • Appropriate volume and/or microphone use
OBSERVER COMMENTS: *STRENGTHS:* *AREAS TO IMPROVE:* SCORE: _____	**OBSERVER COMMENTS:** *STRENGTHS:* *AREAS TO IMPROVE:* SCORE: _____
III. VISUAL AIDS (Check all that apply) • Color palette and design were cohesive • Effective data visualization • Font was legible • Images were clear, relevant and culturally sensitive • Slides were not cluttered; presentation was visually engaging	**IV. RESPONSE TO QUESTIONS** (Check all that apply) • Tone in response was constructive (not defensive or argumentative) • Presenter(s) fully answered questions • All team members participated in responding to questions • Responses were professional and ethical • Overall, presenter(s) anticipated questions well
OBSERVER COMMENTS: *STRENGTHS:* *AREAS TO IMPROVE:* SCORE: _____	**OBSERVER COMMENTS:** *STRENGTHS:* *AREAS TO IMPROVE:* SCORE: _____
Total Score:	
ADDITIONAL NOTES	

■ ACT ACTIVITY 7

Actually give the presentation, with others role playing being the attendees at the presentation meeting. Video your presentation and evaluate it as a team using the evaluation tool provided in this chapter.

REFERENCE

1. The Visual Communication Guy. *The Rhetorical Appeals*. 2019. https://thevisualcommunicationguy.com/rhetoric-overview/the-rhetorical-appeals-rhetorical-triangle

CHAPTER 15

PRACTICE ACT STEP A3: IMPLEMENTATION AND MONITORING

ACT STEP A3: IMPLEMENTATION AND MONITORING

As shown in Figure 15.1, there are two substeps in the Implementation and Monitoring step in the Act phase of the Problem-Solving Method: A3.1, Develop a detailed implementation plan; and A3.2, Monitor results against key performance indicators.

Remember to go back to Chapter 2 to read the "what" of Step A3 before starting the practice of the "how" in this chapter.

Step A3 often involves active involvement of personnel from other parts of the organization; for example, the performance improvement or project management department. Although you will need to develop and provide the detailed implementation plan and metrics to be monitored for your recommendations, you will not likely have the authority to assign organizational resources to carry out the implementation plan or metrics monitoring.

PRACTICE A3.1: DEVELOP A DETAILED IMPLEMENTATION PLAN

A detailed implementation plan delineates all of the tasks that need to be carried out to implement the recommendations, along with the time frame, the deliverables, the deadlines, the personnel and financial resources, and the responsible "owners" of the tasks and the overall plan.

HOW TO DEVELOP A DETAILED IMPLEMENTATION PLAN

Too often, managers think that a problem has been solved once consensus has been developed or a recommendation has been accepted with an action plan. But the best recommendations will not fix the problem if they are not implemented. Once your recommendations have been accepted, they must be enacted.

Actual implementation is much more difficult than identifying the key milestones in Act step A1.2. Implementation of change is a complicated process, involving the full

ACT

A1. Recommendations & Milestones	A2. Communication Strategy & Consensus Building	A3. Implementation & Monitoring
A1.1 Create integrated set of _recommendations_ A1.2 Develop key implementation milestones	A2.1 Revisit stakeholder analysis A2.2 Create communication plan A2.3 Implement communication plan and validate approval/consensus of recommendations	A3.1 Develop detailed implementation plan A3.2 Monitor results against key performance indicators

FIGURE 15.1 Act step A3: Implementation and monitoring.

range of technical, interpersonal, social, and other skills. Nonetheless, that change process must still occur, and it is often the healthcare leader's role to energize that change process.

As you gain experience, you will develop a better understanding of how big of a change is required in the organization to implement potential alternative solutions, and how that may impact the probability of success. This would factor into your decision-making process as a decision criteria during the Study phase.

It is not the intent of this section to go into great detail about the process of implementation and change. The important message here is that the problem-solving process must produce results, and results can only be assessed once the recommendations have been successfully implemented.

For student consulting projects, and for case competitions, you usually do not get into the detail of a complete implementation plan. Usually your work in terms of implementation detail stops at the level of the key milestones. If the organization is requesting a detailed implementation plan, it should be stated in your scope of work document.

KEY STEPS TO DEVELOP A DETAILED IMPLEMENTATION PLAN

Step 1: Review the key recommendation milestones created in Act step 1.2.

Step 2: Create work streams for each key recommendation. Develop accountabilities and goals for each work stream. Charge each work stream with a first task of developing a detailed implementation plan.

Step 3: Collaborate with the organization's project management personnel to identify the appropriate staff to include as team members in the implementation process.

Step 4: Create, with teams, detailed project plans for each major milestone.

TIPS TO DEVELOP A DETAILED IMPLEMENTATION PLAN

- Many organizations have a preferred project management approach. Before creating details, check with the organization to see if there are internal project managers and/or project management technology platforms that the organization uses, and incorporate the details of the plan into these formats and/or tools.

TOOLS TO DEVELOP A DETAILED IMPLEMENTATION PLAN

Project management software is used to create a detailed implementation plans. Microsoft Project is an example of project management software.

ACTIVITIES TO DEVELOP A DETAILED IMPLEMENTATION PLAN

◼ ACT ACTIVITY 8

Build out a detailed implementation plan for one key milestones in Act step A1.2

PRACTICE A3.2: MONITOR RESULTS AGAINST KEY PERFORMANCE INDICATORS

Key performance indicators are metrics that are tracked to help the organization understand if the recommendations have solved the problem as defined. They arise from the goals identified from your issue statements and problem statement, and from the decision criteria you developed in Study step S2.1 to evaluate alternative solutions.

HOW TO MONITOR RESULTS AGAINST KEY PERFORMANCE INDICATORS

In the short run, a monitoring program of some sort, be it formal or informal, should always be a part of the manager's mindset relative to a specific change. In the long run, the manager and the organization must recognize that evaluation of the effectiveness of the organization, either related to specific questions or in a very broad sense, is a responsibility that one must consciously apply in the problem-solving thought process.

In this sense, the problem-solving thought process is not only applicable to problem-oriented situations, but it is also a process consciously applied when a problem or situation is not evident. This often occurs through a monitoring process whereby the organization consciously assesses its own performance. These feedback loops are a critical component of a systems approach to problem-solving.

In student consulting projects, and in case competitions, you should always present a set of key performance indicators that the organization should track to know if the recommendations are working as intended. You should also specify the target for which the organization should be striving on the indicators.

KEY STEPS TO MONITOR RESULTS AGAINST KEY PERFORMANCE INDICATORS

Step 1: Review the key recommendation milestones created in Act step A1.2.

Step 2: Review any goals in your issue statements and problem statement, and review the decision criteria developed in Study step S2.1.

Step 3: Develop key performance indicators for the entire set of recommendations, using your goals and decision criteria as a guide.

Step 3: Set key performance indicators for any of the milestones or specific recommendations that will need special attention paid as if not met, as they would put the organization and/or project at risk.

Step 4: Establish a plan for monitoring and reporting on the key performance indicators, including who is responsible for monitoring the key performance indicators.

TIPS TO MONITOR RESULTS AGAINST KEY PERFORMANCE INDICATORS

- Understand the organization's strategic goals and how they are measuring success. Look to articulate how the benefits of your proposal add to the success of the goals and measurement already established in the organization. This is important to do before you would create new metrics, as there is time and money involved in creating new ways to measure success.

- Not all metrics are "forever" metrics. Determine if this is a short-term indicator that is needed to understand if a threshold is being met, or if the metric needs to be tracked ongoing.

- Understand and research the difference and connection between the lead and lag indicators.

- If a new metric needs to be tracked, before suggesting the indicator, ensure you have met with finance or IT to establish that it is feasible to collect the data necessary to track the metric.

TOOL TO MONITOR RESULTS AGAINST KEY PERFORMANCE INDICATORS

Most organizations have computerized tools or dashboards they use to track performance.

ACTIVITIES TO MONITOR RESULTS AGAINST KEY PERFORMANCE INDICATORS

■ ACT ACTIVITY 9

For one of your recommendations, identify a key performance indicator and a target to which the organization should be striving.

MAKING THE PROBLEM-SOLVING METHOD AUTOMATIC

Congratulations! You have learned and practiced all of the steps and substeps of the Problem-Solving Method. We encourage you to work through additional cases provided in Part V of this text to provide you with more practice. It is through practice that the Problem-Solving Method becomes the way your brain naturally thinks when you are faced with problems.

There are a variety of ways you can use the cases. If you want to practice the Define phase only, you can work through several of the cases only through the point of the last step of the Define phase—the problem statement and vision for the future. If you want to complete all the steps of the Problem-Solving Method, we recommend you focus on a couple of cases only, especially because the Problem Study phase can be time consuming to do it right. And, as you practice, you should write out the steps.

Remember that in real life, for any given problem you face, you will not be using every single step and substep every single time. Whether the problem you are facing is a three-minute conversation in the hallway or a months-long complex situation, you will have internalized the "never assume" mindset, and you will be able to quickly think through problems in real-time to identify the difficulties and key issues that need addressing, with an approach to study and act to resolve the problem.

Never assume.

CHAPTER 16

ACT PHASE ACTIVITY KEY

A1.1: CREATE INTEGRATED SET OF RECOMMENDATIONS (IN CHAPTER 13)

■ ACT ACTIVITY 1 KEY

Review your set of recommendations for The Spinal Frontier. Decide on a category that will effectively help explain the recommendations in an integrated set. Arrange the recommendations by this category. Add any additional recommendations that are missing from your analysis and arrange these in the category. As a reminder, categories to consider are by timeline (e.g., short-term vs. long-term), importance, stakeholder, and any others you can determine.

One approach would be to organize the recommendations by timeline, as shown in Table 16.1.

■ ACT ACTIVITY 2 KEY

Think ahead to the presentation strategy step. What visuals or frameworks come to mind when looking at the recommendations as a whole? Review diagrammer.com or PowerPoint SmartArt to see if any frameworks come to mind.

Figure 16.1 shows an example of an approach for visualizing the key milestones of the recommendations.

A1.2: DEVELOP KEY IMPLEMENTATION MILESTONES (IN CHAPTER 13)

■ ACT ACTIVITY 3 KEY

Create a Gantt chart of the key milestones for your The Spinal Frontier recommendations. Remember to focus on the major milestones and not on implementation detail.

Figure 16.2 provides an example Gantt chart for the key milestones.

TABLE 16.1 Spinal Frontier Recommendations Organized by Timeline

SHORT-TERM	MID-TERM	LONG-TERM
Prism Health should proceed with the joint venture to establish a MedSpine program at Westport Hospital	The structure and role of the Prism Musculoskeletal Clinical Service Line (PMSCSL) needs to be re-defined	Prism Health should approach Prism Health Plan and create a Spine Center of Excellence
The steering group should have authority and should include directors from Neurosurgery, Orthopedics, Sports Medicine, Physical Therapy, Occupational Therapy	In the existing world of value-based care PMSCSL should have clear clinical protocols in place to screen and treat patients with spine issues	

Prism - Building the Spine Care Continuum

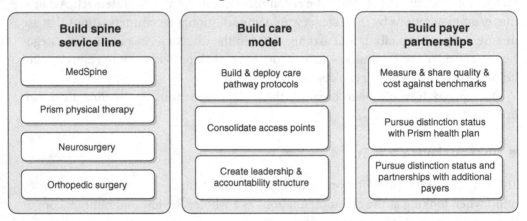

FIGURE 16.1 Spinal Frontier key milestones for recommendations.

A2.1: REVISIT STAKEHOLDER ANALYSIS (IN CHAPTER 14)

■ ACT ACTIVITY 4

Suppose one of your recommendations is to move forward with the MedSpine joint venture.

Which stakeholders might be opposed to that recommendation?

What scenario or contingency might you put in place to what end?

Table 16.2 provides examples of some of the key stakeholders' concerns about the joint venture and your proposed contingency plan.

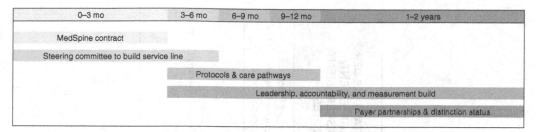

0–3 mo	3–6 mo	6–9 mo	9–12 mo	1–2 years

MedSpine contract

Steering committee to build service line

Protocols & care pathways

Leadership, accountability, and measurement build

Payer partnerships & distinction status

FIGURE 16.2 Spinal frontier key milestones Gantt chart.

A2.2: CREATE THE COMMUNICATION PLAN (IN CHAPTER 14)

■ **ACT ACTIVITY 5 KEY**

Table 16.3 shows an example communication plan for The Spinal Frontier project preceptors, who are also the Musculoskeletal Clinical Service Line dyad leaders, and the Musculoskeletal Clinical Service Line steering committee.

A2.3: IMPLEMENT THE COMMUNICATION PLAN AND VALIDATE APPROVAL/CONSENSUS OF RECOMMENDATIONS (IN CHAPTER 14)

■ **ACT ACTIVITY 6 KEY**

Prepare a PowerPoint presentation for Prism Health System. Those attending will be your preceptors (the Dyad leadership team of the Musculoskeletal Clinical Service Line), the CEO and COO of Prism Health System, the CEO of the Prism Health Plan, the hospital CFO, the Spine Surgeon, the Director of Physical Therapy, and others on the Musculoskeletal Clinical Service Line advisory group.

TABLE 16.2 Stakeholder Concerns and Contingency Plan

STAKEHOLDER	POSSIBLE DISAGREEMENT	PLAN
Physical Therapy Director	Will be concerned about the MedSpine decision	Meet with PT Director to discuss plan and how the partnership is a complement, not a competitor
Hospital CFO	Will be concerned that additive costs will not have a payback and surgeries will decline	Discuss pro forma with CFO and review assumptions on capturing, overall more patients

TABLE 16.3 Example Communication Plan for Preceptors and Steering Committee

GOALS	DESCRIPTION & DETAILS OF FORUM + ATTENDEES	WHAT IS THE KEY FOCUS FOR THE AUDIENCE	IN WHAT FORMAT WILL THE INFORMATION BE COMMUNICATED	WHO WILL COMMUNICATE THE INFORMATION	STAKEHOLDER AGREEMENT/ DISCERNMENT NOTES
Project Preceptor	Prep meeting before the Steering Committee in their office	Review draft of plan and presentation	PowerPoint draft document with Appendix	Project Manager of team to send 48 hours before meeting	Project Preceptor concerned about CFO's reaction
Steering Committee	Monthly Steering Committee meeting. In Board Room with U shaped table, technology available, lunch served, presenters usually stand	Plan approval via consensus, group does not take a formal vote	PowerPoint draft document with Appendix. Supplemental pro forma in Excel	Project Manager will send PowerPoint to administrator 5 business days ahead of meeting for pre-read. CFO to receive pro forma 5 days ahead from Preceptor	CFO and Physical Therapy Director concerns

Review your presentation and ask yourself the following questions:

- Does your presentation contain the elements of Aristotle's Rhetorical Triangle—Logos, Ethos, and Pathos?

- Does your presentation tell a compelling story with a clear beginning, middle, and end?

- Have you designed your slides to be engaging and compelling and visually interesting to look at?

- Is it clear from your slides where you are in the presentation?

- Have you made sure to avoid problem-solving "lingo" in the presentation?

- Are you finishing your presentation with a clear call to action?

- Have you anticipated questions that might be asked by your audience and how you will answer them?

■ ACT ACTIVITY 7 KEY

Actually give the presentation, with others role playing being the attendees at the presentation meeting. Video your presentation and evaluate it as a team using the evaluation tool provided in Exhibit 14.1 in Chapter 14.

Public speaking is a very anxiety provoking activity for many people. Yet it is a key leadership competency.

As you engage in critiquing your presentation, consider the following:

- Learn how to both give and receive constructive feedback about your presentation style and areas for improvement in presentation skills. Use the example presentation criteria provided in Chapter 14 to guide your discussions.

- As you watch your presentation, look for the following:

    - Do you display confidence and enthusiasm for what you are presenting?

    - Are you maintaining eye contact with your audience? Or are you turning your back to them and talking to the screen? Are you reading your presentation, or are you speaking in a conversational manner? Are you using a lot of "filler words" such as "um," "ah," or "like"?

    - Are you using the room to your advantage, or are you hiding behind the podium? Are you hiding your hands under the table? Hiding your hands behind your back? Crossing your arms in front of your body? Are you wiggling in your chair? Are you engaging in any other annoying behaviors because you are nervous? If so, you need to become consciously aware of these habits so that you can stop them.

    - Are you confident when answering questions? Are you getting to the point of your answer or rambling? If presenting with a team, are you sharing the question answering, or is one of you dominating and not letting the others have a turn?

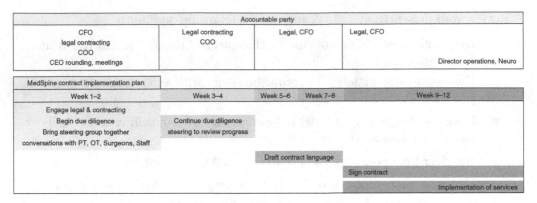

FIGURE 16.3 MedSpine contract implementation plan.

A3.1: DEVELOP DETAILED IMPLEMENTATION PLAN (IN CHAPTER 15)

◼ ACT ACTIVITY 8

Build out a detailed implementation plan for one key milestone in Act step A1.2

Figure 16.3 provides an example of a Gantt chart that identified the detailed steps required for implementing the MedSpine contract.

A3.2: MONITOR RESULTS AGAINST KEY PERFORMANCE INDICATORS (IN CHAPTER 15)

◼ ACT ACTIVITY 9

For one of your recommendations, identify a key performance indicator and a target to which the organization should be striving.

Example MedSpine Key Performance Indicators

- Number of new non-surgical spine patients served increases by 50%
- Days to be seen for initial evaluation reduced by 10%

PART V

PROBLEM-SOLVING CASES

OVERVIEW OF PART V

Part V of the text has 14 cases to provide you with opportunities to practice the Problem-Solving Method. The cases are arranged in four chapters. As stated in earlier chapters of the text, you should write out each of the steps when practicing the Problem-Solving Method. This helps you learn how to internalize the steps, such that it becomes the way your brain automatically approaches problems you will face in your career as a healthcare leader.

Chapter 17 provides you with five cases that are operations and quality focused. For those of you with minimal healthcare experience, these cases might be easier for you to grasp compared to cases that are more strategic in nature. Operations and quality cases generally have a focus that is more internal to the organization compared to cases that are more strategic in nature.

The five cases in Chapter 18 focus on strategic issues. Cases involving strategy require you to focus both internally in the organization, as well as analyze the external environment to determine the best course of action. In doing so, you assess the strengths, weaknesses, opportunities, and threats to the organization as part of your problem-solving process.

Chapter 19 provides two cases that focus on population health. These two cases are longer in length than those in the other case chapters. They address social determinants of health that are challenging healthcare systems to engage in broader community collaboration to resolve societal issues that result in poor outcomes related to health and well-being. Although you can work through these cases on your own, they are particularly well-suited to be solved by teams whose backgrounds span multiple professions, including health, housing, social services, and so on.

Chapter 20 provides two cases that focus on long-term care. The first case in Chapter 20 is operationally focused. The second focuses on a strategic issue in long-term care and aging services in healthcare organizations.

When you read a case, there may be terms or situations that may be unfamiliar to you. For example, one of the operations cases addresses a situation of nursing Magnet status. Before working through the case, you may need to do some preliminary research and come to an understanding of what Magnet status is, how it is achieved, and why an organization would pursue Magnet status. This provides you with skills in searching out preliminary information for topics on which you are not well informed. Part of becoming an effective leader is learning how to learn.

You can practice the Problem-Solving Method in a number of ways, depending on what you are trying to master. If you want to practice the Define phase steps, you can work through a number of cases focusing on just the steps of that phase. If you want to practice how to study a problem through doing research, then pick the cases in which you are most interested in learning about the topic depicted in them, and work through both the Define and Study phases. If you wish to gain experience in presenting, then work through the case in its entirety, and engage with others in doing mock presentations.

At the University of Minnesota's problem-solving course, a case is assigned to a team of students. During the semester, the students complete two cases—the first is an operations-based case such as those in Chapter 17, and the second is a strategy-oriented case such as those in Chapter 18. The students have several weeks to work through the case to provide ample time for conducting the research for the Study phase of the Problem-Solving Method.

You will see that all of the cases in Chapters 17, 18, and 20 indicate the role that you are in the organization (e.g., you are the CEO, or you are the VP, or you are the Chief Nursing Officer). To provide students in the problem-solving course with practice in thinking through presentation strategy and gaining experience in presenting, the students then role-play the case. Each person in the case presentation group has a different case. The students present their own case, and also role play the stakeholders in the other cases when they are not the ones presenting. The typical format is for a student to present, followed by questions from their fellow role-playing students.

You will also see that in many of the cases, you are asked to present to a group. In some cases, it is the leadership team of the organization. In other cases, it is the board of directors. These two groups have very different responsibilities in the organization. Leadership team meetings will be more operationally and detail focused. The decision-making is typically through consensus, not formal voting.

By design, boards of directors focus on strategic issues because they are the governance body or the organization. As such, the information they receive should be more strategically oriented, rather than providing operational detail. Boards should not be involved in the daily operations or operational structure of the organization. That is what they hire the CEO. Healthcare organization boards do expect updates from the CEO when something has happened in the organization that is affecting the organization's reputation in the community or threatens the sustainability of the organization. Board decision-making is generally formal; for example, following Robert's Rules of Order[1] when conducting the meeting, and taking formal votes for courses of action recommended by the CEO. If you role-play cases in which the presentation is to the Board, one of the group members should take on the role as Board Chair.

If you have never attended a leadership team meeting you should ask your mentor if you can attend a meeting in their organization. If you are in a summer residency or your fellowship, you should take the opportunity to attend as many of the leadership team meetings as you can. To see how board meetings function, you can also attend an open meeting of a public board, such as for a university, or watch a city or county board meeting which is often shown on the local cable channel. Also, ask for permission to attend the board meetings during your summer residency or fellowship so that you gain an understanding of how boards function and their role in organizational governance of healthcare organizations.

Finally, whether you are a member of a student project team, a summer intern or resident, a fellow, or further in your healthcare career, you do not have to be in a positional authority leadership role to demonstrate leadership. Leadership is a competency and mindset that is required from all levels of authority in the organization. Becoming a "never assume" problem solver will support you throughout your career.

REFERENCE

1. Price N. *Robert's Rules of Order Cheat Sheet for Nonprofits*. Board Effect (blog). 2018. https://www.boardeffect.com/blog/roberts-rules-of-order-cheat-sheet

CHAPTER 17

OPERATIONS AND QUALITY CASES

OVERVIEW OF OPERATIONS AND QUALITY CASES

Operational and quality situations often have one or more issues that need immediate resolution, in addition to longer-term issues that need to be addressed to fix the system that allowed the situation to occur. The analogy is that a patient suffering a heart attack will require immediate treatment followed by long-term health behavior change to prevent another occurrence.

Thus, when addressing these types of situations, you will need to ensure that you pay attention to the prioritization of your recommendations. Be sure that your recommendations address the immediate, the short-term, and the long-term when warranted.

In operations and quality cases, it is also important that you engage in the "never assume" mindset that requires you to engage in self-reflection to identify if you are part of the problem.

Finally, although we recommend using humor in presentations where appropriate, it is not appropriate to make light of the situation when a serious error has occurred that has harmed a patient. Additionally, taking care in what handouts or materials are utilized in the presentation is very important due to patient and staff confidentiality.

CASE 17.1: NUTRITION SERVICES AT MEMORIAL HOSPITAL

You are the VP for support services at Memorial Hospital. The Nutrition Services Department reports to you. You just received the last quarter's Patient Satisfaction and Quality results; for the fourth quarter in a row, patient satisfaction with food service has decreased. One comment in particular struck you: "When did you start serving ice-water soup?" Additionally, the quality report shows a significant increase over the past 6 months of meals served to NPO patients and late meal arrivals for diabetic patients. No adverse events have been reported, although a handful of cases were marked by physicians and nurses as "near misses" in the quality database.

You recall that your last conversations about this subject with the Nutrition Services Director was 2 months ago; she said budget and staffing cuts are hurting her department's performance. Since then you have cut another $80,000 from the department's budget to help the hospital meet the system's profit goals.

Memorial has a monthly meeting of the Quality and Patient Satisfaction Improvement Team. This team consists of the other VPs and key department heads and is chaired by the Chief Operating Officer. The Nutrition Department near misses and patient satisfaction and quality results are an agenda item for the group at its meeting next week.

What will you report and recommend?

CASE 17.2: BLOOD TRANSFUSION ERROR AT SANGUITO HOSPITAL

You are the CEO of Sanguito Hospital, a large regional medical center in an East Coast city. A female patient was admitted to your facility to give birth. The OBGYN ordered blood work for the patient and entered the order in a computerized order entry system and utilized the lab bar coding system. The patient had a blood sample tested to identify the blood that may be needed in the event of a complication. Later in the afternoon, the female patient had complications after giving birth and needed multiple blood transfusions.

Around the same time, a male patient arrived in the emergency department suffering from multiple gunshot wounds. He was rushed into an adjacent trauma OR due to the severity of his injuries. A blood sample was sent to the lab to complete an analysis and testing. The male patient lost quite a bit of blood and many transfusions were needed during his procedure; therefore, the patient care assistant (PCA) had to make multiple trips to the blood bank.

When the female patient needed additional blood for the transfusion, an order was sent to the blood bank, where the blood was issued to a different PCA. However, due to the hectic afternoon in the OR and the need for multiple blood products, a hallway exchange occurred between PCAs. After the exchange, a PCA began carrying the blood for the two patients to "save time," which is against protocol.

The PCA dropped off the cooler containing the female blood product in the male trauma patient's room and then dropped off the other cooler with the male's blood product in the female's operating room. In a hurry, the staff transfused the male blood without inspecting the paperwork or looking at the female patient's wristband. Minutes later the error was realized and the blood bank was alerted prior to the utilization of the incorrect blood for the male patient. This was difficult to sort out in the chaos, although it was determined that the male did not receive the wrong blood as the OR staff was able to identify the wrong sample and avoid transfusing.

The error resulted in an adverse event where the female patient died. You were in your office when you received a call from the surgical suite notifying you that a major quality event occurred and that a patient died. In following up with the nurse unit manager and blood bank manager, you have learned that the patient care assistants, the anesthesiologists, and both care teams involved are devastated by the error.

In accordance with your hospital's policy, you joined the surgeon and Patient Representative to meet with the family of the woman who died and the male trauma patient's family to inform them of the error. You expressed your sincere condolences to the families and offer your assistance helping them through this difficult time.

The following day, you received a call from a local reporter requesting a comment on the incident. While you did not disclose the incident to the media, it is not uncommon for the media to find out when a patient medical error and/or death occurs.

At this point, you are uncertain if the families plan to file a lawsuit against the hospital or the physicians, but you need to be prepared for that contingency. A meeting with the Board has been scheduled for later this week for you to discuss an action plan to respond to this event. In addition to addressing the public relations and liability issues resulting from this situation, the Board chair has asked you to share how you plan to ensure that similar incidents are prevented in the future. What will you present to the Board?

CASE 17.3: EBOLA AT REVERE COMMUNITY MEDICAL CENTER

It is the fall of 2014, and you are the CEO of Revere Community Medical Center, a large tertiary care center in a major metropolitan area. Early this morning, you received a call from the Chief of Emergency that a patient that arrived via ambulance meets initial screening for Ebola. The Chief reports to you that the patient is in isolation, the State Department of Health has been notified, and they are on their way to the facility to collect samples for testing. The State Department of Health has contacted the Centers for Disease Control and Prevention (CDC) to inform them that there is a potential positive at your facility. If diagnosed as positive, this will be the first case of Ebola diagnosed in the United States.

You also receive a report from the Medical Chief of Emergency Medicine that, according to the family and the medical record, the patient visited the hospital's emergency department (ED) 3 days ago and was discharged. The Medical Chief indicates that after reviewing the record, he learned that the patient presented with a low grade fever and was discharged from the ED with antibiotics. According to the Medical Chief, it is noted that the patient recently traveled to the United States from an area of the world with a growing number of Ebola diagnoses, although the information was "buried" in the past medical history section of the electronic chart and was not obvious at the time of the previous ED visit, according to the attending ED physician who cared for the patient earlier in the week.

You learn that a command center has not been established and call the emergency preparedness manager to immediately initiate a command center with the CNO, CMO, Directors of Infection Control, Patient Safety, Employee Health, and Emergency Management.

Throughout the day and evening you receive the following information:

The patient has tested positive for Ebola.

The Nurses' Union president reports to the Chief Nursing Officer (CNO) that they will likely file a complaint, as nurses are reporting that not all the Personal Protective Equipment (PPE) covers the neck area of staff members as recommended by the CDC. The Union president said and the CNO agrees that it appears that the guidelines in Emergency Management are not being followed and that things seem "chaotic." Despite union concerns, many physicians, nurses, and other staff are calling to offer to work extra hours if needed.

The patient's family has called Patient Relations, insisting that the new experimental drug to fight Ebola become available to their family members. They are threatening to initiate litigation if the hospital does not comply.

Additionally, the local and national media are calling your office to inquire about a possible "Ebola patient" and the previous visit of the patient to the ED.

The Director of Surgical Services indicates that patients are calling to cancel surgeries and families/patients are starting to ask questions.

The Chair of the Board of Directors has called a special Board meeting for tomorrow evening and has asked you to present a short-term action plan and to outline long-term considerations.

CASE 17.4: DRUG DIVERSION AT RIVER VALLEY HOSPITAL

River Valley Hospital is a large, tertiary care center located in downtown River Valley, California, a city with a population of 300,000. It is the largest hospital in the River Valley area, and has a reputation regionally for its high quality care.

You are the VP with responsibilities for surgical services, having been in this position for the last 5 years. Your director of surgical services is relatively new to her position, having been with the hospital for 4 months. The previous director had been in this position for 15 years prior to her retirement 4 months ago. The new director commented to you that she is working hard to try to reduce the high nurse staff turnover rate she inherited in surgical services and is worried about a nursing shortage in the area that seems to be most acute with nurse anesthetists.

The director came to you late this morning with a problem for which she said she needs help.

Earlier this morning, a male patient was undergoing a kidney stone procedure under local anesthesia. The urologist and the staff involved in the procedure came to the director immediately after the procedure with some disturbing news. They reported that the patient was in so much pain during the procedure that the staff had to hold him down to finish the procedure. During the procedure the urologist repeatedly asked the nurse anesthetist who had given the patient his pre-op pain medications to get back to her patient and figure out why the pain meds he had ordered and that she had given him before the procedure started weren't working. The urologist and staff reported that the nurse anesthetist slurred her words and seemed unsteady on her feet.

After receiving this news, the director approached the nurse anesthetist in question, and found empty syringes with the labels peeled off in the pocket of her scrubs. This is a violation of hospital policy. The director has mandated a drug test of the nurse anesthetist, which came back positive for the narcotic pain medication that was supposed to have been administered to the patient. She also talked with the patient after he had recovered enough from surgery to speak. The patient reported to her that the nurse anesthetist told him prior to his surgery that he would have to "be a man" to take the pain he was going to feel during the procedure, because they couldn't give him a lot of pain medication. The patient is furious, and is threatening to sue the hospital.

You did some investigating and learned that the nurse anesthetist in question had jobs in two other entities of the hospital, including the ambulatory surgical center and the affiliated children's hospital in the past 5 years. The nurse anesthetist started working in this OR 3 months ago and was transferred to this unit following staff complaints. You remember learning that there is a nurse anesthetist shortage in your state.

You informed your CEO of the incident and what you have learned. He is asking for a meeting at the end of the day with the leadership team and the director of surgical services for your plan of action. What will you recommend to the leadership team?

CASE 17.5: MAGNET STATUS AT HEARTFIELD MEDICAL CENTER

In March, you were appointed Chief Nursing Officer of Heartfield Medical Center and have been in your position for 3 weeks. Heartfield Medical Center is the flagship 400-bed hospital of the Heartfield Health System located in downtown Nassau, a city with a population of 350,000. Shortly after leading your previous hospital, Lutheran Valley Hospital to Magnet status, you were aggressively recruited by Heartfield with the objective of the hospital being re-recognized as a Magnet hospital. Re-recognition occurs every 4 years and for Heartfield it will occur in the beginning of the next calendar year.

Given that Heartfield's nursing and medical staff weren't nearly as large as Lutheran Valley's, you made the assumption that the job wouldn't be as challenging as the first time around, since Heartfield is currently a Magnet hospital. After a few short conversations with the other executives at the hospital when you started in March, you felt confident Heartfield would be ready by the end of the year, giving you 9 months to prepare.

You immediately assembled a team and began conducting a SWOT analysis of the nursing staff to identify their strengths, but more importantly their weaknesses and possible opportunities and threats that needed to be addressed if Heartfield is to be successful in this effort. After approximately 3 weeks of data collection and informational interviews with staff nurses, nurse managers, other staff, and physicians, the findings suggest that things are much worse than you had initially realized. You are concerned Heartfield will not pass recertification and that a strike could be on the horizon. The area of concern is centered on "performance improvement on measure TL1 (nurse practice environment), which includes nurse satisfaction, nurse turnover rates, productivity, and nurse-assessed quality of care."

Your meetings revealed that an overwhelming majority of the staff nurses felt as if Heartfield is a top-down organization where their thoughts are not valued. More specifically, they felt as if they do not have enough involvement in the decision-making process of patient care delivery and staff ratios. In addition, interviews reveal that nurses believe Heartfield physicians are not open to true collaboration, are difficult to work with, and not respectful of nurses. You also found that there is not a sense of open communication among all nurses, and even worse communication between nurses and other members of the health care team.

Additionally, you found that there are differing philosophies among nurses of differing specialties and job classes, and many are uninformed of the hospital's patient outcomes percentile rank.

In reviewing employee satisfaction survey data, you find that more than 60% of the nursing staff reported having a low level of job satisfaction. Additionally, in the month of February and March there were reports of increased union meetings and activity, which could result in upward of 800 of Heartfield nurses going on strike.

The interviews with the nurses seem to correlate with the 33% turnover rate for bedside RNs at Heartland. This high rate also nudged you to look into variables such as compensation and work environment. You found out that salaries and fringe benefits are well below the state's average and last year there was a change to health benefits, with nurses now having deductible-only options, where in the past, there was still an "affordable" plan to which there was no need to meet a deductible before 100% coverage. With what seemed like a lack of passion for their jobs and distrust of nursing leaders and executive management, it is not difficult to see why the nursing culture at Heartfield seems so stagnant. Many of the physicians revealed that in their opinions, nurses at Heartfield had a "union level mentality."

You have your work cut out for you if you are to have Heartfield Medical Center "Magnet-ready" in 9 months and to address a possible strike. You have a meeting in 1 week with the rest of the Heartfield leadership team. They are expecting updates on your findings, any implications that they may have, and a short-term and long-term action plan. What are you going to discuss and recommend?

CHAPTER 18

STRATEGIC HEALTHCARE CASES

OVERVIEW OF STRATEGIC HEALTHCARE CASES

At its core, strategy is answering these three questions: (a) where is our organization now; (b) where do we want it to be in the marketplace given our organization's strengths, weaknesses, opportunities, and threats, often referred to as a SWOT analysis; and (c) how do we get there. There are situations in which both operational and strategic issues must be addressed simultaneously, therefore you shouldn't think that situations you face in your career are going to be either operational or strategic. Your role as a leader is to balance both, or to be ambidextrous.

Strategy issues require focusing both internally and externally to the organization. As a leader, you need to engage in environmental scanning to ensure your organization is successful both now and in the future. In healthcare, positioning the organization strategically for success often entails partnering or merging with other organizations or entities. Joint ventures are an example, where two or more organizations maintain their separate identities, while jointly partnering in a commercial endeavor. In mergers, the entities do not remain as separate organizations.

If you research strategic planning processes, you will see that there are many similarities to the Problem-Solving Method, except that the focus is on strategic planning. Table 18.1 shows how they are similar:

TABLE 18.1 Similarities Between Strategic Planning and the Problem-Solving Method

STRATEGIC PLANNING	PROBLEM SOLVING METHOD
Conduct an Internal and External Analysis	Uncovering Difficulties
Articulate Mission, Vision, Values of the Organization	Vision for the Future
Identify Critical Areas and Pillars	Problem Areas
Goals	Decision Criteria
Tactics	Recommendations

CASE 18.1: WESTRIDGE HOSPITAL SYSTEM INTEGRATION

You are the CEO of Westridge Hospital, a 30-bed rural hospital in Iowa. There is a primary care group attached to the hospital, with six family practice physicians, two internists, and a pediatrician. The hospital has done well historically, has adequate reserves, and is planning a $5 million remodeling project to upgrade its facilities.

About 8 months ago, as the project was being planned, you heard the clinic was planning to add some laboratory and radiology services, which would shift revenue from the hospital to the clinic. To get ahead of this movement, you proposed to the clinic CEO and administrator that the hospital and the clinic be merged. They agreed to explore this possibility, and it has been studied productively for the past several months.

Agreement has been reached on a broad range of issues. The structure agreed upon is one in which the clinic and hospital employees will become employees of a newly integrated system, and all non-professional fee income (hospital and clinic) will be pooled. The doctors will have a separate but closely affiliated practice. There will be a new Board for the newly integrated system with a governance structure with four out of nine Board members being physicians. The organization will operate in the market as one system, with agreed upon economic parameters. All of this has, to date, been agreeable to the clinic, the hospital Board, and yourself. Even the attorneys have reviewed the proposals and have signed off.

But there is now a disagreement over leadership of the newly integrated system. You thought there was agreement on a management model in which you would become the CEO, the clinic administrator would manage the outpatient activities of the system, and the hospital management team would manage the inpatient operations. However, at last week's hospital Board meeting, one of the physicians (Dr. Wilson) proposed a co-CEO arrangement, so that there would be "appropriate physician leadership in our newly integrated system." According to Dr. Wilson, who is a hospital Board member, the issue of physician leadership is a deal-breaker for the physicians. One of your Board members (Mr. Clauser, a local feed store businessman) agreed, saying he had discussed this with his doctor at the clinic at the time of his last exam. Mr. Clauser also said it does not seem that the physicians trust you, the CEO.

The discussion last month deteriorated quickly, and the Board chair cut it off by asking you to prepare a set of recommendations for management of the new system for next month's Board meeting.

When you returned to your office from the Board meeting, three of your senior managers came to see you. They expressed concern about the physician leadership model. They also said that some of the departmental reporting relationships that are being envisioned in the new system are not appropriate. The Director of Nursing feels the ER and the clinic nurses should report to her, instead of the clinic administrator. The VP of Support Services feels Medical Records and Quality Improvement should continue to report to him.

What will your recommendations at the Board meeting be?

CASE 18.2: HOPE HOSPITAL JOINT VENTURE

You are the CEO of Hope Hospital, one of three hospitals in a city in the Northeast. The three hospitals are highly competitive, as you would expect, especially in a time of declining inpatient utilization. None of the three hospitals has a significant edge on the other two, in terms of market share or reputation.

Hope has a significant emphasis on Orthopedics, and has a high quality reputation for its progressive Ortho program. Hope started a joint venture 1 month ago with Century Ortho, one of the predominant Ortho groups in the market. This joint venture is intended to be a high quality, high value (lower cost) option for certain Orthopedic patients who need surgery, but whose immediate post-op care can be delivered in a non-hospital setting. This joint venture, which operates down the block from the hospital and uses a hotel across the street, is called OrthoQual.

OrthoQual, as a 50/50 joint venture, is governed by a seven-person Board: three from the Ortho group (Century Ortho), three from Hope, and a community representative. The joint venture has a management agreement with Century Ortho to manage the operations of OrthoQual. The OrthoQual Executive Director is Sheila Rasmussen, who was previously the Clinic Manager of one of Century Ortho's clinic sites. Hope's Ortho Service Line Executive, Mary Marshall, MHA, is the lead liaison from Hope to OrthoQual. Through 1 month of operations, it is clear to Mary that Sheila is in over her head. When Mary brought up the potential of bundled payments, Sheila did not even appear to understand what they are.

You were in your office last Monday morning when there was a knock on your door. You recognized someone who is a casual acquaintance, who is also someone who is well known and well respected in the healthcare community and beyond—Marla Wilkins, RN, PhD. Dr. Wilkins is a Professor of Nursing at the local state university. She was obviously very upset as she told you the story about the recent care of her sister at OrthoQual.

Dr. Wilkins indicated that she has asked her sister, Brenda Greeley (who is a CPA partner in a local accounting firm), if she could speak to officials at Hope about the care she (Ms. Greeley) received at OrthoQual, and Ms. Greeley consented.

Ms. Greeley (the patient) is a 50-year-old female with a history of cerebral vascular accident (CVA) with left side weakness, but no cognitive or verbal limitations, compromised aortic valve (secondary to subacute bacterial endocarditis), and seizure disorder (secondary to CVA). She is cared for through her primary care physician and her neurologist, both of whom are part of the employed physician group at Hope.

Over the last 2 years her left foot has been contracting inwardly due to left side nerve involvement from the CVA. The patient was referred to an orthopedic physician whose subspecialty is complex foot care. The orthopod, James Robertson, is part of Century Ortho.

Dr. Robertson recommended surgical repair of the patient's left foot, with the surgery to be done at OrthoQual. The patient concurred. She went through the pre-op physical, including blood work and EKG from her primary care physician.

Following a successful surgical repair in the Ambulatory Surgery Center (ASC) at OrthoQual, the patient was transferred to the hotel where the patients stay after surgery in the ASC. Nursing staff from OrthoQual provide care and care coordination.

Upon discharge from the ASC, and transfer to the hotel setting, the discharging nurse was heard (by the patient's husband) saying to colleagues, "who is this patient's doctor and how does he like to handle these stays?"

When the patient arrived at the hotel room she was interviewed by another nurse, who asked, "what medications is she on?" The PA who works with the surgeon had provided pain management orders for the stay.

The nurse explained that the medications supplied for the one night stay will "not exactly be the same" as what the patient usually takes; generics will be used. When the husband asked "why," the nurse said, "we are trying to be a low cost provider here, and generic drugs are less expensive."

Both the patient and the husband forgot to report the seizure medication to the nurse.

The patient had a difficult night. The husband had gone home at the patient's urging at about 9:00 pm. In the early hours of the morning, his wife called him in tears because she was experiencing significant pain. His wife told him that the nurse would only give her Tylenol with codeine for pain. His wife requested additional pain meds, and was told by the nurse that "she didn't like to give that medication if the patient was to be discharged the next morning, and was not supposed to give it in the hotel setting." Later it was discovered that the PA working with the surgeon had also prescribed Patient Controlled Analgesia for the patient to administer pain meds, thinking the patient was going to be admitted to the hospital for the one-night stay. This order was not followed.

When the husband arrived in the morning he was, of course, very upset, and asked to speak with a manager. He did so, and was told, "our team will discuss this and get back to you."

The patient was discharged to home the following morning in severe pain with little or no sleep following surgery. The patient took a full dose of oral pain medication at home, but severe pain persists. She does not recall if she took her received seizure medication while in the hospital. She experienced a "breakthrough" seizure; the first in 8 months. This event has consequences for the patient's lifestyle for the next 6 months, as the seizure is a reportable event requiring total driving restriction.

The primary care physician had called the patient's home the day after surgery, because he could not access the medical record at OrthoQual and could not reach the Orthopedic Surgeon. When the patient returned 5 days post-op for her visit with the Orthopod, he was unaware of everything that had transpired post-op.

At the time of Dr. Wilkins (the patient's sister) visit with you, it is 10 days post-op and the family had still not heard anything from OrthoQual in follow-up to the events following surgery and the concerns expressed by the husband.

You are very concerned about what you heard about this patient's care from Dr. Wilkins. You asked Mary Marshall to look into the case. Mary and Sheila Rasmussen gathered a report the same day; it basically confirmed the report you received from Dr. Wilkins. When you reviewed the report you asked about quality and safety protocols that have been developed at OrthoQual. Ms. Rasmussen's response was, to the effect of "we are so new we are still working on those things."

Mary pulled you aside after the meeting and expressed her concern about Sheila and if the joint venture could be successful under her management. She pointed to this event and the fact that limited data on the financial and quality/patient experience has been shared to date. Mary added that surgeons visiting OrthoQual have also expressed concern over the joint venture.

There is a meeting of the OrthoQual Board tomorrow evening. You are on the Board, and intend to bring this matter up (respecting patient confidentiality) at the Board meeting.

What will your course of action include, both at the Board meeting and in follow up to what you have heard?

CASE 18.3: STRATEGIC INVESTMENTS AT WALLACE HOSPITAL

You are the CEO of Wallace Hospital, a Critical Access Hospital in the Upper Midwest. Wallace has been on a positive trajectory over the past several years. Six new primary care physicians have been recruited; two Orthopedic Surgeons, a General Surgeon, and a Urologist have also established successful full-time practices. These are all hospital-employed physicians, as are several other primary care physicians at Wallace. You and the Board at Wallace decided years ago to go in the physician employment direction, largely because the other primary care practice in town, which is a satellite clinic of All Angels, a large system an hour away, was not focusing its efforts on this clinic, which caused the clinic to stop growing. The All Angels practice, which once consisted of 8 primary care physicians, is now down to 4, with two more retirements likely in the next few years.

Inpatient and outpatient volumes at Wallace are up 12% over the past 3 years. Financial performance has been positive (4% operating margin), and a previously depleted balance sheet now has 180 days cash on hand. The inpatient facilities at Wallace however are out of date, with only double rooms, which is not consistent with today's standards. There are other facility deficiencies as well. You have a preliminary estimate of $30 million for a facility update from an architectural firm. Your accounting/financial advisory firm indicates that if positive performance continues you will be in a position to finance a project of that scope and support the related debt service.

Three events/pieces of information are causing you to pause, however.

The first is that there is a rumor that All Angels is planning to pay more attention to its satellite clinics in general and in your community specifically, including an addition to the local clinic to do more outpatient procedures, therapy, and imaging work.

The second is the recent emergence of limited network health plan products in the state. These products are health system/insurance company joint ventures. Wallace has already been excluded from one such limited network plan; however, the product offered by the health plan has only nominal presence in the market. The other new plan is co-owned by All Angels and a large national insurance company (All Saints), and they have announced a major marketing effort. The provider network for this new product ("Signature") will be oriented around the All Angels facilities and providers.

The third is an annual report from a quasi-state agency that was produced last week. This report compares cost and utilization performance of primary care groups (and, indirectly, their related hospitals). Wallace is measured at 19% above the state cost average on a case-mix, risk adjusted basis. This report is publicly available and is in the line of sight of the health plans in the state. Your immediate reaction is one of concern: If we are 19% above the norm, we will not be an attractive provider for limited network products.

The report indicates that the 19% variance is driven by above-average utilization and above-average prices, each making up half of the given variance (9.5% each). The immediate reaction of the physicians at Wallace is that the utilization data are wrong. The first reaction from the CFO is that we have negotiated successfully for our rates, and that has been part of our financial success, which is enabling us to consider the $30 million facility upgrade project.

You are scheduled to bring the $30 million project for final Board approval next month. There is a high level of medical staff, employees, Board, and community support and excitement for the project. What will your recommendations and plans be, especially in light of the more recent market developments and comparative data?

CASE 18.4: COMMUNITY CHRONIC CARE IN HARRIS, ALABAMA

You are the CEO of Harris Community Hospital, a 200-bed private, not-for-profit acute care facility located in Harris, Alabama. It is the only hospital in the county, and hence has virtually all the market share for the county, as well as a large market share for an additional six surrounding counties that are primarily rural agricultural. As CEO, you recognize that the market is moving to paying for outcomes, not for process. Medicare has implemented reimbursement changes for certain diseases to improve the quality of hospital care and incent more coordinated care post-hospitalization. It has changed its reimbursement policies for excess readmissions within 30 days for patients who were hospitalized for conditions such as heart attack, heart failure, and pneumonia, and soon will be changing its reimbursement policies for patients with chronic obstructive pulmonary disease, coronary artery bypass graft, percutaneous transluminal coronary angioplasty, and other vascular conditions who are readmitted within 30 days.

Furthermore, the Institute for Healthcare Improvement's articulates the need for a "Quadruple Aim" approach to health system redesign to provide safe, effective, and efficient care, especially to patients with chronic disease. They articulate four dimensions of performance that must be pursued simultaneously:

- Improve the patient experience of care, including quality and satisfaction;
- Improve the health of populations;
- Reduce the per capita cost of healthcare; and
- Improve the work life of healthcare providers.

The organizational models of physician practices in your community make these changes especially challenging. There are nearly 200 physicians spanning 30 specialties with practice privileges at the hospital. The hospitalists and emergency medicine physicians are employed by the hospital. The other physicians are distributed among many independent practice groups across the community.

For example, the two allergist/immunologists have their own small practice, as do the four dermatologists and the four ear, nose, and throat specialists. The 24 family medicine physicians are spread among six practice groups, with two of the practice groups having six physicians each. Ten of the 12 internal medicine physicians are spread across two practice groups in the community, with the remaining two practicing in small towns in the adjoining county. The two internal medicine physicians that also provide geriatric specialization are split between the two practice groups in the community. There is one pulmonologist in the community with a solo practice, Dr. Diaz. His two other partners recently left the practice for other professional opportunities. With only one pulmonologist in the community, the lead time for a pulmonary outpatient appointment is 4 weeks. All of the physician groups have their own medical records systems, none of which interface with each other or the hospital's Epic electronic medical records system.

Harris Community Hospital does not own nor operate any home health or post-acute care services. There are 11 nursing homes in the area, with Medicare's nursing home compare website showing widely disparate rankings in quality among them. There are five senior living communities, some of which offer assisted living in their continuum of care. Home health services are provided by the county, while hospice care is provided by a small not-for-profit company that has a 15-bed hospice facility.

As you look at this fragmented system of healthcare services in the community, you believe it is a core driver of your organization's poor performance in meeting national care guidelines. Of immediate concern, Harris's 30-day readmission rates for primary or secondary COPD is almost 25%. A large proportion of these patients are being admitted with either a primary ICD diagnosis of COPD, or a secondary diagnosis of COPD underlying a primary diagnosis of pneumonia. National guidelines for COPD care indicate that spirometry should be performed annually. It is estimated that only 20% of patients with COPD in the community are meeting that guideline.

While patients with COPD are in the hospital, nurses educate them on the correct self-management techniques to use their nebulizer equipment and minimize COPD exacerbations. If the patient looks like they are having difficulties, the respiratory therapist from the hospital will make a home visit soon after the patient is discharged to ensure they are using their nebulizer properly. They will also help order and set up oxygen therapy if needed.

The social workers in the hospital may also determine that the county home care services should make intermittent or regular visits to ensure the patient is continuing their self-therapy and following up with their physician. With only one pulmonologist in the community, the majority of COPD care is provided by the patient's primary care physician. On consultation, Dr. Diaz will see COPD patients in the hospital or verbally confer with the hospitalist to determine needed therapy changes. After being discharged, patients will then follow up with their own physician and discharge summaries are emailed to that physician. Dr. Diaz will see patients in the outpatient setting who are referred to him by the patient's primary care physician for consultation.

This story of care is similar for chronic disease care generally in the community. The hospital staff may be providing some of the care, the county may be providing home care services, patients are being seen by their primary care physicians and being referred to specialists as needed, and the patient and family are trying as best they can to coordinate care on their own. The irony is that your hospital is in some sense "rewarded" every time an admission occurs, since it generates revenue, although the reimbursement is changing for some readmissions within 30 days. However, in the meantime, trying to do the right thing by improving the care in the community may in many cases result in reduced reimbursement to the hospital if admissions decrease.

At the end of your last Board meeting, one of your Board members described the saga of his father's care over the past 6 months for his COPD and congestive heart failure, going in and out of the hospital 3 times before finally being admitted to a nursing home after his most recent hospital discharge. He described the poor quality of life for his father, the stress on the family, and his father's adjustment at not being in his own home anymore.

This led to a discussion of the challenges already described, and how other organizations have been responding to them. The Board has asked you to come to a Board meeting in 2 months with a plan for how Harris Hospital should move forward in addressing the fragmented care system that exists in the community, and how the solution will address the challenges in providing value, while at the same time remaining financially healthy as an organization.

CASE 18.5: NEUROSERVICES AT HARTVIEW HEALTH SYSTEM

Hartview Health System comprises three hospitals and 15 clinics located throughout the western metro region of Hartsville. The system leadership team comprises the System CEO, three Operational VPs, and the CFO. You are one of the three Operational VPs, with administrative responsibilities for running Wegman Hospital. The other two Operational VPs each have administrative responsibilities for running their respective hospital in the system, Albion Hospital and Fenway Hospital.

Although there are two other competing health systems that each have a hospital located in this market, Hartview has maintained a strong market penetration for not only its primary market area, but also for patients in smaller communities farther to the west who come to Hartview for more complex neurovascular and neuro-oncology care at Wegman Hospital.

Hartview Health System's medical staff comprises both employed physicians and independent physician groups. Historically, the employed physicians have tended to be primary care physicians, with the specialists belonging to independent medical groups who have privileges to practice at your hospitals and your competitors' hospitals. However, in the past few years, Hartview has begun employing a small number of specialists.

These employed specialists tend to have subspecialty practices, which enables them to "push the envelope" in providing highly specialized care in a narrow range of disease states with better clinical outcomes (e.g., treating neurovascular disease as opposed to broader neuro disease states). This has created relationship tensions and turf issues with other specialists practicing at Hartview, whose practices still resemble a "generalist specialist" approach to medical care that was more common over the past 20 years than now. In the "generalist specialist" model, a specialist does not subspecialize in particular procedures within their area of specialization.

Five years ago, Hartview made a major several million dollar capital investment in stereotactic radiosurgery technology for Wegman Hospital. The system recruited a neurovascular surgeon, and hired as employed physicians vascular neurologists and neuro intensivists. The neurovascular surgeon has a significant neuro administrative role at Wegman, spending approximately 2 FTE (full-time equivalents) of time in this role.

In addition to the stereotactic radiosurgery technology, the system made a variety of other capital infrastructure investments at Wegman Hospital for highly specialized neuro services, including a neuro ICU with critical care nurses highly skilled in caring for complex neuro patients, ORs with the best capabilities, and two neuro biplane angiography suites. Hartview also invested in telemedicine capabilities to enable access to the best stroke specialist expertise in the health system regardless of which of the system's hospitals a patient is admitted. These investments have increased the volume of specialized neuro cases treated by Wegman Hospital from both its primary service area and referral area.

As these investments were made, the System CEO indicated to you that Wegman Hospital would be the provider of tertiary care for neurosciences services in the Hartview System. Unfortunately, there was never a frank discussion among the system leadership team (the CEO, the three Operational VPs, and the CFO) of the strategic implications of this decision, namely that the other two hospitals would remain community hospitals and not develop tertiary level neuro services. This has created friction with the other two Operations VPs, who have expressed negative comments about Wegman "getting all the neuro procedure cases."

Based on the success in developing the neurovascular subspecialty program and its growing volume referral stream, the system wants to develop other neuro subspecialty lines that can leverage the strengths and investments the system has already made. The Hartview CEO has charged you with developing a neuroscience service line strategy for the system. He also has asked you to investigate what other specialties besides neurovascular might best utilize the technological capabilities at Wegman Hospital, and if and how those specialties should be pursued.

This has intensified friction with the two other Operational VPs, who view this as something that will only help Wegman Hospital, and probably at the expense of their hospitals. They have also made comments that if the clinical lead for a neuroscience service line is the neurovascular surgeon, they will fight it. Although the vascular neurosurgeon has exceptional specialist expertise and is revered by his patients, their families, and the collaborating referring physicians, some of the other Hartview physician leaders and the Operational VPs have complained that he is very arrogant.

As you think about a strategy for developing a neuroscience service line, you recognize that the number of general neurosurgeons practicing at Hartview hospitals has declined over the years. This has primarily been because as the independent practices to which these neurosurgeons belonged experienced retirements, there was no succession planning within the group practices. There are still two independent neurosurgeon groups in the area with highly successful, busy practices, although the groups perform very few of their surgical procedures at Hartview facilities. The other general neurosurgeon groups are employed by the competing health systems across the metro area.

As you build a neuroscience service line, you ponder whether you should buy either or both of the remaining neurosurgeon groups, hire your own neurosurgeons, or contract with the employed neurosurgeons of other systems. You recognize that other large independent specialty groups, such as the large independent orthopedic practice, have appreciated that you are the only system in the area that hasn't employed large numbers of specialists. These groups worry that if your system moves in that direction, then Hartview will redirect spine surgery referrals away from the independent orthopedic surgeons.

The CEO has asked you to come to the system leadership meeting in 3 weeks with your recommendations around a strategy for building and implementing the neuroscience service line and for other specialty areas the system should pursue to fully leverage the investments in its neuro technological capabilities.

CHAPTER 19

POPULATION HEALTH CASES

OVERVIEW OF POPULATION HEALTH CASES

The following two population health cases have a different format than the others. They are longer and address complex issues that are broader than what you typically think of as "healthcare" cases. They are included because, as a healthcare leader, you have a responsibility beyond your organization to improve the health of your community. Social determinants of health, such as poverty, health disparities, and homelessness, are drivers of poor health outcomes.[1]

Improving the health of populations requires that healthcare organizations move "upstream" to address social determinants of health. However, healthcare organizations cannot do this alone. Population health improvement entails healthcare organizations partnering with other sectors with whom they have not traditionally partnered.[2,3] Thus, successful healthcare organizations are both well-run, effective organizations internally, *and* they are partners with other sectors in the community, such as housing, transportation, social services, and public health, in moving upstream to improve the health of the community.

The two population health cases are used with permission of the case writers and CLARION, a University of Minnesota interprofessional student organization that hosts a national case competition. They are especially instructive for interprofessional teams of students.

CASE 19.1: HOME IS WHERE THE HEALTH IS

This case is reprinted with the permission of CLARION at the University of Minnesota, and the case authors, Justine Mishek, MHA, Carolina De La Rosa Mateo, Samantha Shipley, Victoria Smith, and Donald Uden, PharmD, FCCP, at the University of Minnesota. © 2019 University of Minnesota Board of Regents.

■ THE SETTING

In 2017, the U.S. Department of Housing and Urban Development estimated that on any given night, almost 540,000 people were experiencing homelessness. About two thirds of those individuals were staying at emergency shelters or transitional housing, and one third were staying in unsheltered locations. While the number of people experiencing homelessness increased by just under 1% between 2016 and 2017, homelessness has declined by more than 83,000 people since 2010, a 13% reduction. The recent increase in homelessness is attributable to an increase in the number of individuals staying in unsheltered locations in major cities.[4]

Hennepin County is the most populated and fastest growing county in Minnesota. Hennepin County and the surrounding Twin Cities area is home to 19 Fortune 500 companies. The county has the second highest median income in Minnesota at $71,000 and has an average age of 36. The median property value in Hennepin County is $257,700, and the homeownership rate is 61.1%. About 10.9% of the households in the county are identified as in poverty, lower than the national average of 14%. Hennepin County has a strong backbone of health and social services and the county is known for a high quality of life. Amid this prosperity, however, there are over 9,300 individuals experiencing homelessness in Minnesota. Almost half of those experiencing homelessness are situated in Hennepin County.[5]

Every 3 years the Wilder Foundation conducts a survey to understand the reality of those experiencing homelessness. The numbers represented in the study show a "single night count" which is considered the most effective way to understand the scope of homelessness within a region. The number fluctuates due to the difficulty recording the number of homeless individuals at any given time. Homelessness counts likely undercount the actual number of individuals experiencing homelessness, because they don't include people who are not found by volunteers or people who have found a temporary place to stay, such as with friends or family. While Wilder counted 9,312 individuals experiencing homelessness in the state of Minnesota in 2015, it estimates that 15,000 are actually homeless on a given night, and 40,000 experience homelessness in a given year.[6]

The following information was gathered in 2015:

■ Forty-five percent of adults experiencing homelessness are on a waiting list for subsidized housing, with an average wait time of 14 months; another 16% were unable to get on a waiting list because the list was closed.

■ The most common reasons adults left their last housing: 36% could not afford it, 33% were evicted, and 30% lost their job or had their hours cut.

- Adults experiencing homelessness had a median income of $535 during the month of the study and could afford an average of $423 per month in rent; however, one in five could not pay anything for rent.

- It is estimated that 40% of individuals experiencing homelessness may qualify for Supplemental Security Income (SSI) and most can apply for Medicaid/MNsure, General Assistance, and SNAP.[7]

- At the time of the study, fair market rent was $796 per month for a one-bedroom apartment in the Twin Cities.

- Sixty-five percent of adult individuals experiencing homelessness report that they would need an efficiency or one-bedroom apartment.

Hennepin County Homeless Numbers by Study Year, Age Group, and Percent Change Between 2012 and 2015

	2009 Study	2012 Study	2015 Study	% Change (2012–2015)
Children (17 and under) with parents	1,356	1,623	1,360	-16%
Unaccompanied minors (17 and under)	56	35	55	+43%
Young adults (18–21)	371	349	200	-22%
Adults (22–54)*	1,965	1,982	1,647	-17%
Older adults (55 and over)	287	327	403	+23%
Total	4,035*	4,316*	3,665*	-15%

*Young adults age 22–24 are included in the "adults" category so that we can compare to data collected in previous studies.

2015 Counts by Hennepin and Ramsey Counties and Sheltered Versus Not in Shelter

	Hennepin County in Shelters	Hennepin County not in Shelters	Total Hennepin County	Ramsey County in Shelters	Ramsey County not in Shelters	Total Ramsey County
Unaccompanied minors (17 and under)	42	13	55	35	17	52
Young adults (18–21)	166	34	200	157	51	208
Young adults (22–24)	135	22	157	80	21	101
Adults (25–54)	1,320	170	1,490	583	112	695
Older adults (55 and over)	353	50	403	170	20	190

	Hennepin County in Shelters	Hennepin County not in Shelters	Total Hennepin County	Ramsey County in Shelters	Ramsey County not in Shelters	Total Ramsey County
Children (17 and under) with parents	1,350	10	1,360	499	42	541
Total	3,366	299	3,665	1,524	263	1,787

There are multiple shelters in Minneapolis that work to provide transitional and permanent housing. Coordinated Entry is Hennepin County's current system used by shelters and case workers to determine the eligibility and prioritization of housing needs.[8] There are 22 shelters listed on homelessshelterdirectory.com.[9] There are additional shelters in the area, including shelters in various churches, such as First Covenant Church, and self-organized encampments.[10] Each shelter has different qualifications for gender, age, how long a person can stay (short-term vs. long-term), meals, showers, laundry, Wi-Fi/computers, and storage.

As of 2017, there are 600 beds available, down from 650 in 2016 in the city/county. Most evenings, the 600 beds are full, and many individuals are turned away.[11] There are a variety of resources available to those experiencing homelessness outside of governmental case workers and shelters. For instance, a local charity organization publishes a Handbook of the Streets, and there are support groups like Street Voices of Change.[12,13]

■ THE DILEMMA

A recently developed and growing homeless encampment with over 300 individuals has gained the attention of Hennepin County and City of Minneapolis officials, the media, and various community stakeholders.

The highlighted issues include the lack of temporary and affordable permanent housing and the roadblocks individuals face when trying to access and stay in homeless shelters. Additionally, individuals living in the encampment have experienced numerous health emergencies, some resulting in loss of life, including asthma attacks, seizures, and drug overdoses.[14-16]

The majority of adults experiencing homelessness in Minnesota (83%) have either significant mental or physical illness such as a chronic health condition, a substance abuse disorder, or evidence of a traumatic brain injury; 44% have more than one of those conditions.[17-19]

Sixty percent of adults experiencing homelessness reported a significant mental illness; this includes a diagnosis of at least one of the following:

- Anxiety or panic disorder (42%)
- Major depressive disorder (39%)
- Bipolar disorder (22%)

- Personality disorder such as antisocial or obsessive-compulsive disorder (15%)
- Schizophrenia (7%)
- Other paranoid or delusional disorders (6%)

Fifty-one percent of adults experiencing homelessness have a chronic health condition. The most common reported were high blood pressure (30%), asthma (20%), other respiratory problems (12%), other heart or circulatory problems (11%), and diabetes (9%). One in five (21%) of adults experiencing homelessness has been diagnosed with a substance abuse disorder.[6]

The following cases illustrate individuals experiencing homelessness.

Case 1: AB[20]

AB is a 60-year-old man who grew up in Iowa. As a young boy he witnessed his father abuse alcohol, and his father was unable to keep a job. His father moved out, so he and his sister were raised by his mother. His mother worked two jobs at a fast food restaurant and as wait staff at a local eatery. She barely made enough money to support the family. After high school AB held a variety of jobs, none lasting more than 5 years.

AB was married for 15 years. When his wife died in a tragic automobile accident, he went into a 5-year depression and lost his truck driving job. He would not go into work, or was constantly late to work, so he was fired. He didn't have the energy or interest to look for a new job. He found himself out on the street and has been experiencing homelessness for 10 years. He sleeps in shelters, but hates the noise and restrictive rules, and states that "it feels like a prison." During his years on the street, he has had poor oral hygiene resulting in the loss of four of his front teeth. There are dental services that he has tried to access, but they are booked 4 to 6 months out. He had an appointment to address his dental issues but forgot the date and subsequently was scheduled another 4 months out. Recently, he has had job interviews to clean buildings at night; given his appearance, he had had trouble making a good impression: "When you don't have a vehicle and you're missing teeth, these companies are not going to hire you."

Case 2: CD

CD is a 25-year-old man who grew up in Seattle in a very successful conservative middle-income family of four. In high school, he had a psychotic episode where he was hospitalized and subsequently diagnosed with a bipolar disorder. He began self-medicating by abusing alcohol and cocaine. When his mother confronted him about his drug use, he threatened to hit her and was kicked out of the house. He moved to Minneapolis because he heard that it had good public benefits. He panhandles for money and continues to use drugs.

CD doesn't trust shelters because they require sobriety and have so many rules. CD often experiences paranoia, which is exacerbated when he stays at a shelter—one more reason as to why he does not stay in shelters often. CD "sleeps rough." He has a routine where he will alternate sleeping on trains, buses, or in public places that are open 24 hours a day. "Homelessness is not just in shelters. It's in cars and in people's homes." He spends many days in the public library where he can access public computers. For meals he knows which churches and social service organizations offer meals. This requires him to walk blocks to get a meal.

CD has asthma that occasionally flares, exacerbated by cold weather and the air quality in some of the places he stays. He doesn't trust the health care system, but goes once a year to get his asthma medications, which he receives at a local hospital outpatient pharmacy. He is prescribed rescue and controller inhalers for his asthma, but he only uses his rescue inhaler because it works best for him. Because he has no address and no phone number, his pharmacy can't contact him about his controller inhaler. His rescue inhaler has been stolen in the past, so he hides it to protect it. In one incident, he had a severe asthma attack without his inhaler and had to go to the emergency department.

Case 3: EF[22,23]

EF is a 31-year-old mother with a 15-year-old daughter. EF is originally from Illinois. EF has a learning disability; in high-school she was in special education classes and was frequently mocked by her classmates. She had her daughter at the age of 16. The father of her child was in and out of her life and he was both verbally and physically violent. EF eventually fled with her daughter. Not having a job she found herself homeless. Not knowing where to sleep, she and her daughter bounced back and forth between places to stay. Sometimes they stayed at homeless shelters and sometimes with friends. When staying at a friend's place, EF's daughter was abused by her friend's boyfriend. When it was reported, her daughter was taken away by child protective services for neglect. EF was able to regain custody by attending a domestic violence prevention course. Her daughter has significant "mental scars" from her experience and requires mental health services.

EF has a part-time job that pays her about $400 per month which isn't enough to allow her to afford her own home or apartment. She also receives Minnesota Family Investment Program dollars. Because of her learning disability she has difficulty managing her money.

EF is on a waiting list for affordable housing but the wait time is presently 9 months. The Coordinated Entry System doesn't consider her to be vulnerable because she doesn't have a high enough F-SPDAT score and therefore is not prioritized for housing. She would like to have someone who could help her navigate the system. "Where is the program to get people back into society?"

■ THE ASK AND DELIVERABLE

Heading Home Hennepin is a cross-sector group working to end homelessness in Hennepin County.[23] This cross-sectional group is seeking to generate revolutionary and/or novel solutions to address homelessness and health.[24]

Your charge is to propose to Heading Home Hennepin a new, innovative service or community to address housing insecurity and the healthcare of individuals with chronic health conditions as highlighted in the patient case vignettes. The goal should be to create something new or something that significantly improves the current system. See more information on different types of innovation and the Blue Ocean strategy for inspiration.[25,26]

The proposal will include:

- A description of the new service/community
- A description of the ways your proposal will improve the lives and care of those with chronic health conditions that are housing insecure, particularly the individuals in these cases
- A plan to deploy a pilot (funding, those involved, etc.)
- A plan that involves interprofessional teams, various community stakeholders, and how they would be involved in developing and sustaining the program
- A proposed set of outcome measures to include the impact on individuals and the community
- A 5-year outlook of how your solution would be financially and operationally sustainable
  - Assume a one-time grant of $250,000 for start-up costs and/or operating costs. The project is not limited to $250,000. If proposing a budget of over $250,000, teams must develop other plans to ensure financial sustainability through other sources

In addition to your 20-minute PowerPoint presentation, you are required to provide a one-page executive summary of your solution as outlined in the guidebook. We recommend that you limit background information to no more than 5 minutes of your presentation.

CASE 19.2: A GREAT DIFFERENCE: RACIAL DISPARITIES IN INFANT AND MATERNAL MORTALITY AND MORBIDITY

This case is reprinted with the permission of CLARION at the University of Minnesota, and the case authors, Justine Mishek, MHA, and Donald Uden, PharmD, FCCP, at the University of Minnesota. © 2020 University of Minnesota Board of Regents

■ CURRENT SITUATION

National

Within the last 2 years, a large body of research and media attention was brought to light on the rise in African American disparities in maternal and infant mortality and morbidity rates. African American women are up to three times more likely to die from pregnancy-related causes than White women. Additionally, they are twice as likely to suffer from severe complications during pregnancy and birth.[27-30]

Nationally, racial disparities exist for maternal and infant mortality and morbidity. For example, between 2009 and 2014 in the United States, there were 13.0 deaths per 100,000 live births of non-Hispanic White women compared to 42.4 deaths per 100,000 live births of non-Hispanic Black women.[29] Regarding infants, there are also large racial disparities in mortality rates between White infants (4.9 per 100,000) and African American infants (11.4 per 100,000).[30] These racial disparities exist regardless of income or other socio-economic factors.[31] For comparison, the rate of infant mortality is 5.8 deaths per 1,000 live births in the United States, while the average rate in Organization for Economic Co-operation and Development (OECD) countries is 3.8 infant deaths per 1,000 live births.[28]

Within the research, the discussion and evidence focus around various root causes for disparate maternal and infant outcomes, including racial systemic bias, provider implicit bias, access to care, obstetric care (OB) deserts in rural and urban settings, prenatal care, chronic disease management, and social determinants of health.[29,31-35]

State of Wisconsin

Based on 2017 data, the rate of infant mortality in Wisconsin was 6.3 deaths per 1,000 live births, while the average rate of other states was 5.8 deaths per 1,000 live births.[36] Although the average infant mortality rate was close to the national average, the death rate for infants born to African American mothers was the highest in the nation and was three times that of the rate of White mothers. Infant mortality rates of White infants from 2015 to 2017 was 4.6 and was 15.0 for African American infants.[36]

In the most recent data available from 2006 to 2010, Wisconsin had a maternal mortality rate of 5.9 deaths per 100,000 live births, which was lower than the national rate of 16.0 deaths per 100,000 births. However, the maternal mortality rate for African

American women was five times higher than that of non-Hispanic White women, compared to the national disparity of 3.2 times during the same period.[37]

African American infant mortality rates continue to be of concern in Wisconsin. In January 2018, Wisconsin Public Radio highlighted that the state had the highest infant mortality disparity in the United States.[38] WKOW, a television station covering southeastern Wisconsin, specifically addressed the maternal mortality and morbidity issues in March 2019. WKOW focused on the Wisconsin State Department of Health Services report that stated that, from 2009 to 2013, Wisconsin women had serious health complications during 1 of every 100 deliveries. Moreover, the rate increased by 106% between 2000 and 2014.[39]

Southeastern Wisconsin

Southeastern Wisconsin consists of two large cities, Milwaukee and Madison, and 13 counties (Figure 19.1). The cities and counties follow the state trends, with some of the counties experiencing the worst disparities in the state.[40,41] See Table 19.1 for additional details.

Milwaukee, Wisconsin

Milwaukee has been described as one of the most segregated metropolitan areas in the country.[42,43] One fact commonly referred to when discussing segregation is that, "Milwaukee has the lowest rate of African American suburbanization of any metropolitan area in the country."[42] Disparities in housing are tied to historical housing regulations across southeastern Wisconsin. Researchers at the University of Wisconsin-Madison have determined that "16 of the 18 suburbs of Milwaukee County enacted restrictive housing covenants in the 1940s, many of which remained in effect into the 1960s and 1970s."[43]

Discriminatory housing policies have left Milwaukee significantly segregated, with North Milwaukee being home to mostly African Americans.[42] The impact of segregation has greatly contributed to prominent income and wealth inequalities between Whites and African Americans.[44,45] Racial segregation in itself can determine the social and economic resources available to a particular community. Segregation by income can reduce the quality of education available to a community, given that many school districts are funded by property taxes.[31,46]

Racial disparities in social factors have translated into disparities in health outcomes, including maternal and infant mortality outcomes. A study from Johns Hopkins University highlighted that, "Black infant mortality is higher in very segregated cities,"[41] supporting the notion that historical and systemic racism have directly influenced the death rates of African American mothers and infants. Additionally, Williams and Collins have also concluded that "structural racism may contribute to the persisting racial inequity in infant mortality."[47,48]

WISCONSIN - Counties

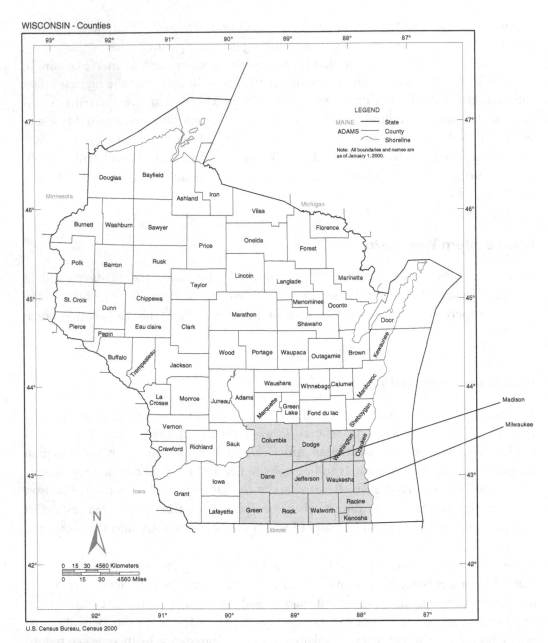

FIGURE 19.1 Map identifying Southeastern Wisconsin focus area.

Source: Original blank map retrieved from https://www2.census.gov/geo/maps/general_ref/stco_outline/cen2k _pgsz/stco_WI.pdf

    The City of Milwaukee has engaged in efforts to highlight racism as a core determinant of health. Additionally, Milwaukee County has declared racism as a public health crisis.[46] Neighborhood revitalization efforts are underway in North Milwaukee, giving local communities opportunities to transform and improve residential life.[44]

TABLE 19.1 INFANT MORTALITY BY COUNTY IN SOUTHEASTER WISCONSIN

	ALL SELECTED	WHITE (NON-HISPANIC)	BLACK/AFRICAN AMERICAN (NON-HISPANIC)	AMERICAN INDIAN/ALASKA NATIVE (NON-HISPANIC)	HISPANIC	LAOTIAN OR HMONG (NON-HISPANIC)	OTHER (NON-HISPANIC)	TWO OR MORE RACES (NON-HISPANIC)
COLUMBIA	5.1	5.3	.	26.3	.	.	.	.
DANE	5.2	4.3	12.8	10.3	4.4	7.6	3.4	12.3
DODGE	5.6	5.7	19.6	21.7	3	.	.	.
GREEN	5.6	5.3	.	.	4.8	X	29.4	.
JEFFERSON	4.5	4.1	22.7	.	3.9	X	9.7	21.7
KENOSHA	5.6	5.1	10.9	11.4	4.6	.	4.5	3.4
MILWAUKEE	8.8	5.2	14.4	8.2	6.1	7.5	5.1	8.5
OZAUKEE	3.7	3.8	10.2	.	.	.	4.2	.
RACINE	8.4	5.9	18.1	9.8	7.5	.	10.2	16
ROCK	6.3	5.5	17.7	13.2	5.3	32.3	6.8	3.1
WALWORTH	5.3	5.6	17.7	.	4	.	.	.
WASHINGTON	4.6	4.5	18.2	16.1	3.3	.	7.5	.
WAUKESHA	4.5	4	11.7	10.2	7.2	.	8.3	.

Source: Data generated from Wisconsin Department of Health Services. WISH (Wisconsin Interactive Statistics on Health) Query: Infant Mortality Module. https://www.dhs.wisconsin.gov/wish/infant-mortality/form.htm

■ MOM AND BABY IN MILWAUKEE[32]

CD is a 34-year-old African American woman who lives in North Milwaukee, Wisconsin, with her two children ages 9 and 11 alongside her husband, RD. She has lived in this area her whole life.

CD is balancing her time owning and operating a local restaurant. CD "grew up" in the restaurant and has enjoyed owning the business since acquiring it from her mother after her dad passed away. CD's husband, RD, is the head chef and assists with operations. CD and RD received a local revitalization grant to update the exterior and interior. The restaurant was featured on a national food show and remains a local favorite. Both CD and RD are very proud to carry the family's tradition forward and look forward to the future.

CD is very involved in her community. She regularly volunteers in the neighborhood revitalization committee when she can, helping others plan and seek funding for their new business ideas.[43] While CD enjoys working and volunteering, she has found it difficult to find the time to add volunteering to her schedule since her mother, JE, moved into her small home after experiencing a life-altering stroke.

The sum of both CD and RD's income from the restaurant does provide for their family's needs. One area of concern in the family's budget, however, is the rising cost of their health insurance. CD and RD purchase their insurance on the individual market, and rising premiums are becoming a budgetary concern. To reduce the monthly cost of health insurance, they moved to a plan with a higher annual family deductible of $8,000.

CD's general health is good, although recently she has been worried about her stress level related to her family and the restaurant. Due to her mom's recent stroke, CD has been tracking her blood pressure on a home monitor she bought at the local pharmacy. CD is concerned that her recent blood pressures are in the 130s/80s range. CD wonders if the added responsibility of taking care of her mother and added household responsibilities--CD's mother used to help keep up with cooking, cleaning, and other household chores--are contributing factors to her elevated blood pressure.

■ EVENT

On Monday morning, while walking her children to the school bus stop, CD began to feel dizzy and nauseated. After her kids were on the bus, she decided that even though she did not feel well, she needed to get to the restaurant for a new staff interview. When she arrived, a server noticed that CD looked like she might be ill and encouraged her to sit down. While she made her way to take a seat, she passed out. The server called 911. By the time the paramedics arrived, she was conscious, and they took her to a nearby hospital. Upon her arrival at the emergency department, providers took her vital signs, medical history, and completed routine lab work including a complete blood count (CBC), comprehensive metabolic panel (CMP), pregnancy test, and a drug screen. During the event, the restaurant staff called her husband, who was running errands for the restaurant. RD arrived at the hospital 15 minutes after CD.

Upon admission to the emergency department, CD's vital signs were: heart rate 90 beats per minute, blood pressure 138/90 mm Hg, and respirations 20 breaths per minute. An

EKG taken in the ambulance on the way to the emergency room did not show any ischemic changes. The emergency department practitioners suspected that her fainting spell was the result of dehydration, and she was administered fluids while laboratory tests were pending. Her laboratory tests revealed that the fainting spell was not the result of dehydration. Her tests also revealed that CD was pregnant. To rule out an ectopic pregnancy, an ultrasound was performed. The fetus was properly placed in the uterus and measured 6 weeks and 2 days. CD was surprised that she was pregnant and pleased to learn the news. It had not occurred to her that she could be pregnant, as her menstrual cycle was not predictable lately. She was advised to follow up with her obstetrician the following week.

After her emergency department visit, CD spent a great deal of time on the phone searching for an appointment that fit her schedule within the health system and office she usually visits. To her dismay, CD had to schedule her 8-week appointment in a different healthcare system in the suburbs, 30 minutes away from her home and restaurant. CD's regular obstetrician switched to Fridays, which is not a good day for her.

At her 8-week obstetrician appointment, vital signs, blood tests, and an ultrasound were performed. It was noted that her blood pressure was 138/83. In response to her blood pressure questions, and after showing her home monitoring results to the obstetrician, they responded, "Well, if you're worried, just make sure to eat healthy, be active—although, don't overdo it, stay off your feet at work, and make sure to sleep."

Over the next several months, CD was able to switch to the clinic closer to her home and continued to attend her monthly appointments. At each appointment, she saw a different provider because the clinic has a team-based care model. Sometimes she was seen by an obstetrician, other times a midwife, sometimes the ultrasound technician, and other times a nurse educator. CD's blood pressure remained elevated in the high 130s/80s throughout her pregnancy, and at each appointment, she asked if she should be concerned. The response from providers consistently was to "just keep your stress and anxiety levels low." She left her appointments discouraged, as she was not confident she could lower her stress or activity with the restaurant responsibilities as well as caring for her mother and children.

At 30 weeks and 5 days gestation, while working at the restaurant, CD developed a headache that would not go away. She tried drinking water, taking acetaminophen, and even taking a nap in the break room, but experienced no relief. Worried that her symptoms may be related to or may impact her pregnancy, she called her obstetrician who advised her to go to OB-triage at the hospital.

When she arrived at OB-triage, on the labor and delivery unit, her blood pressure was 142/90 and her laboratory results showed no changes.

An obstetrics and gynecology intern assessed her and decided that given her age and medical history, they would monitor her for a few hours and give her IV fluids. During their team afternoon rounds, a health professional student on the team asked about CD's blood pressure. The response from the intern was that there was "no concern at this time" and that the patient was "just experiencing anxiety."

Over the next few hours, CD's headache continued as she watched her blood pressure rise. With each set of vitals, she persistently asked about the numbers. Again, she expressed her worry as her mother recently had a stroke, and she had read that sometimes pregnant women with high blood pressure could have strokes. RD also expressed his concern. The nurses called the intern who dismissed RD's concerns and told him that, "there was probably an error with the blood pressure cuff and that it could be changed," and that CD should "take a few deep breaths" and that they "would check again in 10 minutes." CD noticed on the monitor that her blood pressure continued to rise and experienced no headache relief. She was also seeing spots and had blurry vision. CD started to recognize that the provider team seemed to be ignoring her abnormal vital signs and called the nurse multiple times. However, each time, she was told again "not to worry."

The night shift nurse noticed the trend in CD's blood pressure and asked the obstetric attending physician to examine her for chronic hypertension with superimposed preeclampsia. The obstetrician obtained a urine test showing protein confirming the diagnosis and proceeded to prescribe steroids for fetal lung development and magnesium sulfate for neuroprotection. CD was then admitted to labor and delivery for treatment and monitoring.

Over the next few days, the medical team was unable to control CD's blood pressure and decided that the best course of action was to deliver the baby by emergency cesarean section. After an uncomplicated delivery, their baby boy was born and was transferred to the Neonatal Intensive Care Unit. CD and RD's baby was 31 weeks of gestation, and weighed 1,600 grams, making him intrauterine growth restricted. He was intubated at delivery for lack of respiratory effort, placed on a ventilator, administered IV nutrition therapy, and given antibiotics.

Despite successfully delivering the baby, the medical team was still having trouble controlling CD's blood pressure. A few hours post-delivery, she developed sudden weakness in the right side of her face, her mouth began to droop, and she had trouble speaking. Her husband did not understand what she was saying and noticed that she was very confused. He alerted the team who suspected that a stroke might be occurring. They responded immediately by getting an emergent head CT, which showed an ischemic stroke. They administered thrombolytics as soon as possible and halted what they believed could have been a severe stroke.

At 24 hours, the baby's admission blood culture results were positive for a bacterial infection. Despite the Neonatal Intensive Care Unit team's efforts to stabilize him, he developed overwhelming sepsis. After two full code resuscitation attempts, the team was unable to revive him, and CD and RD's baby died at 4 days of life.

While she was able to avoid severe effects of the stroke, CD has some residual right arm weakness and balance problems, which is especially problematic since she is right-handed. She requires ongoing occupational, physical, and emotional therapy. The medical team is very hopeful that she will have a complete recovery, but it may take months for that to occur. CD has a family to think about and care for and a business to operate.

She often asks herself, "Why didn't anyone do anything about my blood pressure? I told them it was high. How will we manage? No one listened to me along the way, and now I have lost my beautiful child."

■ THE MAIN ISSUE AND THE ASK

The bipartisan Black Maternal Health Caucus, a 75-member congressional caucus, aims to "raise awareness within Congress to establish Black maternal health as a national priority, and explore and advocate for effective, evidence-based, culturally-competent policies and best practices for health outcomes for Black mothers."[35] Additionally, an interprofessional organization and collaborative, the Black Mamas Matter Alliance (BMMA) serves as a "national entity working to advance Black maternal health, rights, and justice, and uplifts the work of locally based, Black women–led maternal health initiatives and organizations."[34]

Although national organizations, both the Black Maternal Health Caucus and the BMMA have taken note of the statistics and recent patient stories illuminated by the media in Wisconsin. Additionally, the City of Milwaukee has declared racism as a public health crisis to further acknowledge racial inequities present in Milwaukee.[43,46]

As the Black Maternal Health Caucus and BMMA advocate for change, as the City of Milwaukee illuminates the issues, and as new partnerships are on the horizon, your student consultant team will explore higher African American infant and maternal mortality and morbidity rates. Additionally, your student consulting team will provide recommendations that address those listed in the following.

Your recommendations will be presented as if you are providing the information to a panel of members from the Black Maternal Health Causes, the BMMA, and representatives from the City and County of Milwaukee. The deliverable could include solutions that address policy, community partnerships, community initiatives, and health system initiatives. The deliverable should include the following:

1. A prioritized, innovative set of recommendations to improve the disparities in African American infant and maternal mortalities in southeastern Wisconsin. Additionally, recommendations should address how structural/systemic racism and the history of racial segregation in the United States has impacted the following:

   ■ Systemic racism and implicit bias in healthcare toward African American women in Wisconsin.

   ■ Affordability and access to healthcare coverage and care available to African American women.

   ■ Root cause and solution development in the context of interprofessional management and patient care within hospitals, clinics, and the community.

2. A visionary financing and implementation plan, including:

   a. Estimated costs of the recommendations

   b. Suggested sources of funding

   c. A high-level view of how funding will be allocated

   d. Key performance measures/indicators of success

3. A partnership and accountability plan to drive adoption and sustainability.

In addition to your **20-minute PowerPoint presentation**, you are required to provide a **one-page executive summary** of your solution as outlined in the guidebook.

We recommend that you limit background information to no more than 5 minutes of your presentation.

REFERENCES

1. Begun JW, Potthoff S. Moving upstream in U.S. hospital care toward investments in population health. *J Healthcare Manag.* 2017;62(5):343–353. doi:10.1097/JHM-D-16-00010

2. Kindig DA, Isham G. Population health improvement: a community health business model that engages partners in all sectors. *Front Health Serv Manage.* 2014;30(4):3–20.

3. Noh E, Potthoff S, Begun JW. A taxonomy of hospitals based on partnerships for population health management. *Health Care Manage Rev* [published online ahead of print]. 2018. doi:10.1097/HMR.0000000000000230

4. U.S. Department of Housing and Urban Development. *The 2017 Annual Homeless Assessment Report (AHAR) to Congress.* 2017. https://www.hudexchange.info/resources/documents/2017-AHAR-Part-1.pdf

5. Data USA. *Hennepin County, MN.* 2017. https://datausa.io/profile/geo/hennepin-county-mn

6. Wilder Research. *2015 Minnesota Homeless Study Fact Sheet.* 2015. http://mnhomeless.org/minnesota-homeless-study/reports-and-fact-sheets/2015/2015-homeless-hennepin-county-fact-sheet-12-16.pdf

7. MN Department of Human Services. *Supplemental Nutrition Assistance Program (SNAP).* 2019. https://mn.gov/dhs/people-we-serve/adults/economic-assistance/food-nutrition/programs-and-services/supplemental-nutrition-assistance-program.jsp

8. Hennepin County Government. *Coordinated Entry homeless assistance.* 2017. https://www.hennepin.us/coordinated-entry

9. Homeless Shelter Directory. *Minneapolis Homeless Shelters & Services for the Needy.* 2019. https://www.homelessshelterdirectory.org/cgi-bin/id/city.cgi?city=Minneapolis&state=MN

10. Metropolitan Urban Indian Directors. Franklin/Hiawatha Encampment. 2018. personal interview.

11. Furst R. With too many homeless and too few shelter beds, city funding policy debated. *StarTribune.* 2017. http://www.startribune.com/with-too-many-homeless-and-too-few-shelter-beds-city-funding-policy-debated/445208493

12. St. Stephen's. *Handbook of the Streets Minneapolis 2018-2019: A Resource Guide for People in Need.* 19th ed. 2018. https://ststephensmpls.org/application/files/7815/3900/4312/MHB-1819.pdf

13. Street Voices of Change. Facebook Page. *Downtown Congregations to End Homelessness.* 2018. https://www.facebook.com/SVoC.MN

14. Pember MA. Native homeless woman's tragic death brings light to struggles in Minneapolis. *Indian Country Today.* 2018. https://newsmaven.io/indiancountrytoday/news/native-homeless-woman-s-tragic-death-brings-light-to-struggles-in-minneapolis-9T_oMjcvJUG6hr70gWj_cg

15. Miller P. Second death is linked to Minneapolis homeless encampment. *StarTribune.* 2018. http://www.startribune.com/second-death-linked-to-minneapolis-homeless-encampment/493357271

16. Associated Press. *3rd death linked to Minneapolis homeless encampment. Woman died of apparent overdose.* TwinCities Pioneer Press. 2018. https://www.twincities.com/2018/10/01/3rd-death-linked-to-minneapolis-homeless-encampment

17. Weiss T. People with Disabilities and Homelessness. *Disabled World.* 2017. https://www.disabled-world.com/editorials/political/disability-homeless.php

18. Kaul G. Getting a handle on the size of the homeless population in the Twin Cities. *MinnPost.* 2017. https://www.minnpost.com/politics-policy/2017/08/getting-handle-size-homeless-population-twin-cities

19. Nelson-Dusek S. Start by knowing why: 5 reasons people are homeless in Minnesota. *MinnPost*. 2018. https://www.minnpost.com/community-voices/2018/01/start-knowing-why-5-reasons-people-are-homeless-minnesota

20. Thomas J. The American Way of Dentistry. *Slate*. 2009. http://www.slate.com/articles/life/the_american_way_of_dentistry/2009/10/the_american_way_of_dentistry_3.html

21. World Institute on Disability. *Minnesota Disability Benefits 101*. 2019. https://mn.db101.org

22. OrgCode Consulting Inc. *Family Service Prioritization Decision Assistance Tool (F-SPDAT): Assessment Tool for Families*. Version 2.01. 2015. https://d3n8a8pro7vhmx.cloudfront.net/orgcode/pages/313/attachments/original/1479850993/F-SPDAT-v2.01-Family-Fillable.pdf?1479850993

23. Hennepin County Government. *Heading Home Hennepin Continuum of Care*. 2019. https://www.hennepin.us/headinghomehennepin

24. MN Department of Human Services. *Families and Children Prepaid Medical Assistance Program (PMAP): Health Plan Choices by County*. 2019. https://edocs.dhs.state.mn.us/lfserver/Public/DHS-4324-ENG

25. Satell G. The 4 Types of Innovation and the Problems They Solve. *Harvard Business Review*. 2017. https://hbr.org/2017/06/the-4-types-of-innovation-and-the-problems-they-solve

26. Kim WC, Mauborgne R. *Blue Ocean Strategy*. 2019. https://www.blueoceanstrategy.com

27. Centers for Disease Control and Prevention. *Racial and Ethnic Disparities Continue in Pregnancy-related Deaths*. n.d. https://www.cdc.gov/media/releases/2019/p0905-racial-ethnic-disparities-pregnancy-deaths.html

28. United Health Foundation. Explore Infant Mortality in Wisconsin 2019 Report. n.d. https://www.americashealthrankings.org/explore/annual/measure/IMR/state/WI

29. Centers for Disease Control and Prevention. *Pregnancy Mortality Surveillance System*. n.d. https://www.cdc.gov/reproductivehealth/maternalinfanthealth/pregnancy-mortality-surveillance-system.htm?CDC_AA_refVal=https%3A%2F%2Fwww.cdc.gov%2Freproductivehealth%2Fmaternalinfanthealth%2Fpmss.html#causes

30. Centers for Disease Control and Prevention. *Infant Mortality*. n.d. https://www.cdc.gov/reproductivehealth/maternalinfanthealth/infantmortality.htm

31. Novoa C. *Exploring African Americans' High Maternal and Infant Death Rates*. 2018. https://www.americanprogress.org/issues/early-childhood/reports/2018/02/01/445576/exploring-african-americans-high-maternal-infant-death-rates

32. Office of Disease Prevention and Health Promotion. *Discrimination*. n.d. https://www.healthypeople.gov/2020/topics-objectives/topic/social-determinants-health/interventions-resources/discrimination

33. Center for Reproductive Rights. Research Overview of Maternal Mortality and Morbidity in the United States. n.d. https://www.reproductiverights.org/sites/crr.civicactions.net/files/documents/USPA_MH_TO_ResearchBrief_Final_5.16.pdf

34. Villarosa L. *Why America's Black Mothers and Babies Are in a Life-or-Death Crisis*. 2018. https://www.nytimes.com/2018/04/11/magazine/black-mothers-babies-death-maternal-mortality.html

35. Congresswomen Adams and Underwood Hold Black Maternal Health Caucus Stakeholder Summit. 2019. https://adams.house.gov/media-center/press-releases/congresswomen-adams-and-underwood-hold-black-maternal-health-caucus

36. Wisconsin Department of Health Services, Division of Public Health, Office of Health informatics. *Annual Wisconsin Birth and Infant Mortality Report, 2017 (P-01161-19)*. June 2019.

37. Wisconsin Department of Health Services. *Maternal Mortality and Morbidity, Wisconsin Department of Health Services*. 2019. https://www.dhs.wisconsin.gov/mch/maternal-mortality-and-morbidity.htm

38. Mills S. Wisconsin's Infant Mortality for African-Americans Highest in Nation. *Wisconsin Public Radio*. 2018. https://www.wpr.org/wisconsins-infant-mortality-african-americans-highest-nation

39. Kliese J. Doctors working to address maternal mortality rates in Wisconsin, Mar. 7, 2019. *WKOW*. 2019. https://wkow.com/news/health/2019/03/07/doctors-working-to-address-maternal-mortality-rates-in-wisconsin

40. Downs K. *Why Is Milwaukee so Bad for Black People?* 2015. https://www.npr.org/sections/codeswitch/2015/03/05/390723644/why-is-milwaukee-so-bad-for-black-people

41. Laveist T. *Segregation, Poverty, and Empowerment: Health Consequences for African Americans.* 1993. https://pdfs.semanticscholar.org/ad6b/0d92196eb980a9856c1130cf8ac8871e73b5.pdf

42. Maternowski M. *Measuring Black/White Segregation in Metro Milwaukee.* 2017. https://www.wuwm.com/post/measuring-blackwhite-segregation-metro-milwaukee

43. Maternowski M, Powers J. *How Did Metro Milwaukee Become So Segregated?* 2017. https://www.wuwm.com/post/how-did-metro-milwaukee-become-so-segregated#stream/0

44. Luhrssen D. *Revitalizing North Milwaukee.* 2018. https://shepherdexpress.com/news/features/revitalizing-north-milwaukee/#/questions

45. Pierre J. *Milwaukee Declares Racism a Public Health Crisis.* n.d. https://inequality.org/great-divide/milwaukee-racism-public-health-crisis

46. Branigin A. *Milwaukee County Declares Racism a Public Health Crisis. Will More Cities Follow Suit?* 2019. https://www.theroot.com/milwaukee-county-declares-racism-a-public-health-crisis-1834917218

47. Williams DR, Collins C. Racial residential segregation: a fundamental cause of racial disparities in health. *Public Health Rep.* 2001;116(5):404–416. https://www.ncbi.nlm.nih.gov/pubmed/12042604

48. Wallace M, Crear-Perry J, Richardson L, et al. Separate and unequal: structural racism and infant mortality in the US. *Health Place.* 2017 May;45:140-144. doi:10.1016/j.healthplace.2017.03.012

CHAPTER 20

LONG-TERM CARE CASES

OVERVIEW OF LONG-TERM CARE CASES

The following two cases address leadership issues in long-term care. The first case, Bright Long-Term Care, is operationally based. The second case, Lutheran Care Center, has a strategic focus. Both of the cases will help you develop your knowledge base in the operational and strategic issues that face long-term care organizations.

Increasingly, acute and long term care organizations are partnering to respond to changes in reimbursement for services. Therefore, even if your career is in the acute care sector of the healthcare industry, it is important that you understand the context and environment of the long-term care industry.

CASE 20.1: BRIGHT LONG TERM CARE

You are the administrator of Bright Long-Term Care, a 100 bed long-term care facility. One part of the facility is comprised of five households spread across two floors. The first floor has two households called Green and Red, with 13 residents each. The second floor has three households called Olive, Purple, and Turquoise, also with 13 residents each.

The first floor is staffed with two LPNs and one float CNA, with each household on the first floor staffed with one CNA and one CMA. The second floor is staffed with two LPNs and no float, with two CNAs per household.

The Acuity/MDS levels of the residents on each floor are very different. On the first floor, more than half of the residents can stand by assist or are independent, and only one of the 26 residents requires the use of a mechanical lift. The dependency coding on the first floor is mostly supervision to limited assistance. In contrast, none of the second floor residents are independent, and 28 of the 39 require a mechanical lift or an assistance of two persons. Most residents on the second floor are coded extensive assistance or total dependency.

There is also a large difference in the volume of call lights between the two floors. The second floor has almost twice the number of call lights compared to the first floor. The average call light response times on the second floor had been averaging around 15 minutes, while the average response times on the first floor are about 4 minutes. Residents on the second floor complained to the second floor Charge Nurse 4 months ago about having to wait so long, who in turn immediately talked with the Director of Nursing (DON) about the problem.

The second floor has always had a higher staff turnover rate compared to the first floor. Their annual staff satisfaction survey results have been consistently lower compared to the first floor staff. You received your staff satisfaction survey results 2 months ago, and the results for the second floor staff are the worst they've ever been, even though the first floor looked comparable to past years. You gave the survey results to your DON and told her to take care of it.

One month ago, the DON decided to move the float CNA from the first floor to the second floor. The first floor staff became aware of this change one Monday morning when the first floor Charge Nurse found a yellow sticky note on her computer from the DON. The note instructed the Charge Nurse to send the float to the second floor, because that is where she would be working from now on. When the float nurse appeared upstairs on the second floor to work, the second floor staff was surprised, but very grateful. However, they did complain that the float "didn't know how to lift the residents correctly."

When no education was provided to the float nurse on this issue, one of the CNAs took it upon herself to show the float how she lifts residents.

The first floor staff is very upset. They think it's unfair that the second floor now has more staff than they do when each household has the exact same number of residents. Some of the staff on the first floor have been complaining to their residents about the change. Among the members of the first floor staff that are working diligently, some have complained to their Charge Nurse that some of their first floor co-workers are goofing off and deliberately taking a long time to answer call lights since the staffing change. "This doesn't feel like teamwork" is what one of them reported to the Charge Nurse.

The first floor staff is frustrated that their complaints have not been addressed since this change was made a month ago. You have not been informed by either the DON or the Charge Nurses of any recent staffing complaints at your daily morning operations meetings. You first heard about the rumblings about the first floor this morning, when you got a call from one of the first floor resident's family members, who was very upset about the "attitude and laziness" of the staff on the first floor, and asked if you knew what was going on in your own facility.

After you received the phone call, you emailed the DON, who replied back to you immediately that the staffing change had been very successful. Her reply stated that a month after the staffing change, the call light response times on the second floor had greatly improved, and the average call light response times on the first floor remained the same as before the staffing switch.

Her reply also noted that the staff on the second floor report feeling much less stressed out, and they believe the residents' needs are being better met. She concluded in her email reply by stating that staff on the first floor who are complaining about the decreased staffing level just have a bad attitude.

What will you discuss at tomorrow's morning meeting with the DON and Charge Nurses?

CASE 20.2: LUTHERAN CARE CENTER

This case was written by Leslie Grant, PhD, Emeritus Associate Professor, University of Minnesota. The facts presented in this case are based on actual events but the names and certain details have been changed to protect the identity of the individuals and the organization. Reprinted with permission from the author.

Lutheran Care Center (LCC) provides long-term care services to seniors in the Twin Cities metropolitan area. Its campus is located in St. Paul, Minnesota, and includes a 150-bed nursing home with a transitional care unit (30 beds), an Alzheimer's special care unit (40 beds), and a long stay nursing home (80 beds). The LCC campus has an assisted living facility (90 units), a HUD congregate housing facility (120 units), and a Medicare-certified home health care agency. LCC also provides a variety of senior services through its adult day care center, senior center, and a variety of social services (e.g., Parish Nurse, transportation, caregiver support for Alzheimer's disease, meals program and other services) offered through a network of 46 churches that are part of LCC's corporate partners.

LCC is a faith-based, non-profit corporation that raises about $700,000 per year through fund-raising activities by its foundation to support community-based and other services that are not funded through traditional sources of revenue (e.g., Medicare, Medicaid, insurance or private pay). LCC's mission is to provide high quality services to seniors who are in need based on principles that are grounded in a caring Christian philosophy.

LCC's nursing home has an occupancy rate of about 96%. It has a reputation as a high quality provider and an innovator when it comes to person-centered care. It recently completed a $3.5 million renovation for culture change. However, the campus is land-locked and its buildings (especially the nursing home) could benefit from further renovations. Its most recent application for a moratorium exception for further $5.5 million in capital improvements to the nursing home was not approved by the State of Minnesota. LCC is facing increasing competition from other provider organizations in the Twin Cities metropolitan area—many of whom have relocated their campuses to suburban sites and built brand new state-of-the-art facilities.

The LCC Board of Directors is concerned about the changing market for long-term care services in the Twin Cities metropolitan area. Two issues are paramount:

1. The Twin Cities market has a high penetration rate for managed care organizations that are looking for the "best" providers who can care for enrolled members, including seniors who are being discharged into transitional care units for rehabilitation post-hospitalization. The Twin Cities has three Accountable Care Organizations (ACOs) that are seeking more effective strategies to improve chronic disease management among their members, including seniors living in the community. These ACOs also need to implement systems to decrease the incidence of avoidable hospitalization after discharge to a transitional care unit (TCU). And these ACOs want to enhance chronic disease management of its enrolled members who are living at senior services sites such as LCC campus

(including the nursing home, assisted living facility, congregate housing, and community-based settings).

2. LCC's mission is to serve seniors in need (regardless of the ability to pay). Over the years, the LCC Foundation has provided funds to expand community-ty-based services that help keep seniors out of institutional settings, including LCC's nursing home. Many of these services are not funded by traditional public sector financing programs such as Medicare, Medicaid, and Medicaid Waiver programs. As the need and demand for these services has grown, the LCC Board has asked the CEO and staff of LCC to develop and implement new strategies that make these community-based service programs "sustainable." These programs are targeted to persons with limited income, and they have not generated sufficient revenues to avoid consistent financial losses over the years.

As returns on investment income and money from fundraising activities have become less predictable, the Board has become extremely concerned about the future sustainability of these community-based programs that are operating at a loss. In recent years, these community-based programs have operated at a loss of about $800,000 per year. At the same time, the demand and need for these community-based programs continues to grow. There is a waiting list for these services due to changes in demographics in the Twin Cities metropolitan market, and limited availability of publicly-funded programs aimed at providing community-based services for low-income seniors.

You are the CEO for LCC. You have been asked by the LCC Board to address these two concerns through a new strategic initiative. What will your recommendations be to the Board at its next monthly meeting in 4 weeks?

INDEX

Printed in the United States
by Baker & Taylor Publisher Services

Printed in the United States
by Baker & Taylor Publisher Services